# KETO COOKBOOK

# FOR BEGINNERS

# 2021

50 Easy, Affordable Keto Recipe for
Low-Carb High-Fat Meals Lovers and
Smart People On a Budget.

JENNY BROOKS

# TABLE OF CONTENTS

ZOODLES CARBONARA .................................................................................... 7

LOW-CARB SPAGHETTI BOLOGNESE .......................................................... 9

TURKEY VEGETABLE ..................................................................................... 11

CHICKEN STUFFED AVOCADO ................................................................... 13

EGGS WITH SPINACH ..................................................................................... 15

KETO BREAKFAST SANDWICH ................................................................... 17

INSTANT POT BEEF BOURGUIGNON ........................................................ 20

CRAB STUFFED MUSHROOMS .................................................................... 22

KETO BACON CHEESEBURGER CASSEROLE .......................................... 24

AVOCADO COCONUT ICE CREAM ............................................................ 26

KETO CHOCOLATE MUG CAKE ................................................................. 28

BACON AND EGG CUPS ................................................................................ 30

KETO CHOCOLATE PIE ................................................................................ 31

KETO CREAM CHEESE BROWNIES ........................................................... 33

EASY CHEESY BACON CHICKEN ............................................................... 35

BACON & BRUSSELS SPROUT KEBABS ................................................... 37

KETO ALMOND ROLL ................................................................................... 38

RASPBERRY ICE CREAM .............................................................................. 40

KETO CHOCOLATE DONUTS ..................................................................... 41

KETO FLAN ...................................................................................................... 44

BACON SPINACH DIP .................................................................................... 46

CHEDDAR CHICKEN BREASTS ................................................................... 48

KETO BACON MAC 'N' CHEESE .................................................................. 50

KETO CHOCOLATE CAKE ........................................................................... 53

KETO CAKE WITH CHOCOLATE AVOCADO FROSTING ..................... 55

GLUTEN-FREE CHOCOLATE COCONUT CUPCAKES .......................... 57

KETO RASPBERRY STUFFED CAKE .......................................................... 59

LOW-CARB BANANA PUDDING ................................................................. 61

RASPBERRY LEMON POPSICLES ............................................................... 64

GLUTEN-FREE SPICED KETO COOKIES..................................................................65

CHOCOLATE CHIP KETO COOKIES .....................................................................67

KETO BACONWRAPPED JALAPENO POPPERS .....................................................69

KETO DEVILED EGGS RECIPE WITH AVOCADO AND BACON ...........................71

AVOCADO & EGG FAT BOMBS............................................................................73

KETO ROLLUPS....................................................................................................75

CREAM CHEESE COOKIES....................................................................................77

GRILLED CHEESE SANDWICH .............................................................................79

LOW-CARB BACON JAM .....................................................................................81

BACON "CHIPS" AND GUACAMOLE DIP .............................................................83

AVOCADO EGG SALAD........................................................................................85

KETO AVOCADO TOAST RECIPE WITH PISTACHIO AND TOMATO....................87

TASTY FETA BURGERS (EGG-FREE)......................................................................88

KETO CRACK CHICKEN .......................................................................................89

TOMATO FETA SOUP ...........................................................................................91

LOW CARB GREEN SMOOTHIE ...........................................................................93

KETO PROTEIN SHAKE .......................................................................................94

KETO GREEN SMOOTHIE ....................................................................................95

ANTI-INFLAMMATORY GOLDEN MILK KETO SMOOTHIE...................................97

CINNAMON ALMOND BULLETPROOF KETO SHAKE...........................................99

BUFFALO CHICKEN JALAPENO POPPERS ..........................................................101

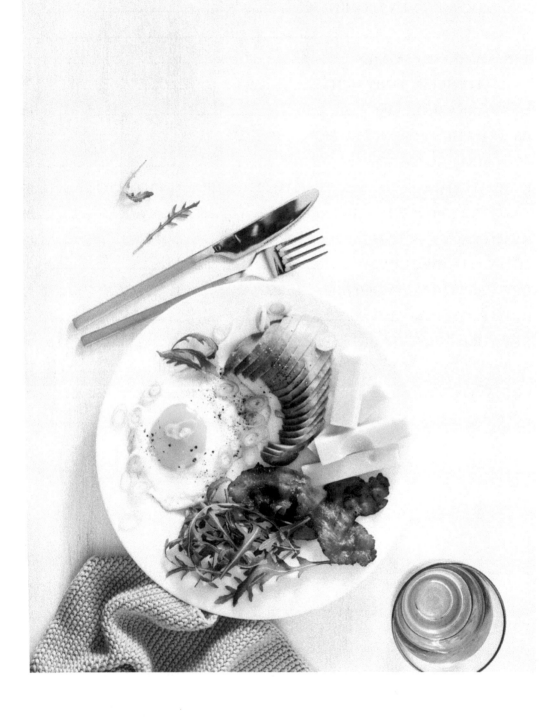

# ZOODLES CARBONARA

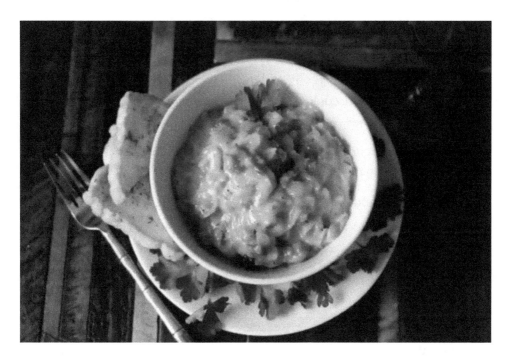

SERVING: 4

**INGREDIENTS:**

2 medium zucchini

8 slices bacon,

Chopped ½ cup onion,

Chopped 1 clove garlic,

Minced 4 eggs

½ cup grated Parmesan cheese

1 pinch salt and black pepper to taste

2 Tbsp fresh parsley

Chopped 2 Tbsp grated Parmesan cheese

## DIRECTIONS:

01. Cut the zucchini into "pasta." If you are using zucchini "pasta" my suggestion is to only serve the sauce on the noodles you will eat that night. The leftover noodles and sauce get a little soggy, so reserve both separate.

02. In a large skillet, cook chopped bacon until slightly crisp; remove and drain onto paper towels. Reserve 2 tablespoons of bacon fat and heat in reused large skillet.

Add chopped onion, and cook over medium heat until onion is translucent. Add minced garlic and peas (if using), and cook for an additional 1 minute.

03. Return cooked bacon to skillet; add cooked and drained spaghetti. Toss to coat and heat through.

04. Add beaten eggs and cook, tossing constantly with tongs or large fork until eggs are barely set. Quickly add 1/2 cup Parmesan cheese, and toss again.

05. Add salt and pepper to taste (remember that bacon and Parmesan are very salty).

06. Serve immediately with chopped parsley sprinkled on top and extra Parmesan cheese at table.

## NUTRITION:

Amount per Serving

Calories 523

Fat 15.5 g

Protein 28 g

Carbs 66.2 g

 Fiber (65.8 effective carbs) 0.8 g

# LOW-CARB SPAGHETTI BOLOGNESE

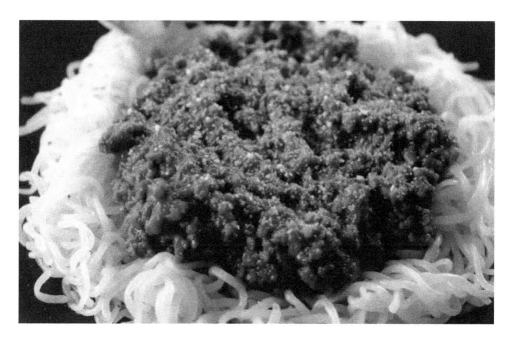

Low-carb spaghetti Bolognese with zoodles is an absolute staple in our house. It can be ready in 20 minutes, start to finish and we always have mince/ground beef and vegetables in the fridge.

SERVING: 5

**INGREDIENTS:**

1 onion finely chopped

2 cloves garlic crushed

500 g mince/ground beef

400 g tinned/canned chopped tomatoes

1 Tbsp dried rosemary

1 Tbsp dried oregano

1 Tbsp dried sage

1 Tbsp dried basil

1 Tbsp dried marjoram salt and pepper to taste

## DIRECTIONS:

01. in a large saucepan. gently fry the onion and garlic in oil until softened but not over cooked.

02. Add the mince/ground beef and continue to fry stirring continuously to break up the mince/ground beef. Fry until all the meat is cooked and browned.

03. Add the herbs, seasoning and tomatoes.

04. Stir then simmer for 15 minutes whilst you make the zoodles. 05. Serve in a bowl with zoodles and grated cheese or parmesan sprinkled on top.

## NUTRITION:

Amount per Serving

Calories 318

Calories from Fat 153

Total Fat 17 g

Total Carbohydrates 13 g

Dietary Fiber 4 g

Sugars 7 g

Protein 30 g

# TURKEY VEGETABLE

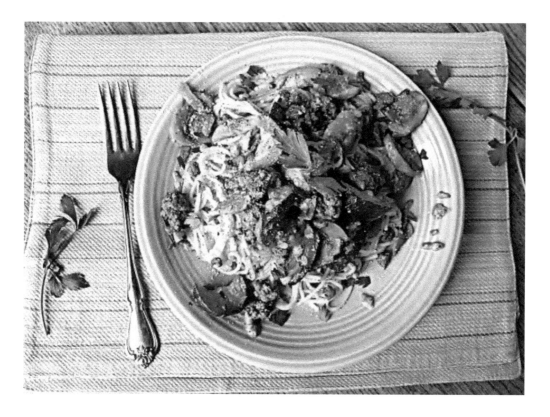

Fresh vegetables like zucchini, mushrooms and onions make for the perfect combination with ground turkey and Homemade Pesto Sauce over pasta.

SERVING: 6

**INGREDIENTS:**

2 tsp oil

1-¼ pound ground turkey

1 cup diced onion

2 cups sliced zucchini

2 cups sliced mushrooms

3 Tbsp Homemade Pesto Sauce

Optional toppings: fresh chopped parsley, grated Parmesan

## DIRECTIONS:

Heat oil in a large skillet and brown ground turkey. Once cooked remove and set aside. Add onion and saute until translucent, then add zucchini and mushrooms. Cook for about 5-8 minutes or until vegetables are tender. Add ground turkey back into pan with vegetables and stir in pesto sauce, cover and lower heat. Simmer 5 minutes.

## NUTRITION:

Calories per serving 273.5

Fat 14.5 g

Cholesterol 76.6 mg

Sodium 126.6 mg

Carbs 5 g

Fiber 1.2 g

Sugars 2.2 g

Protein 20.6

# CHICKEN STUFFED AVOCADO

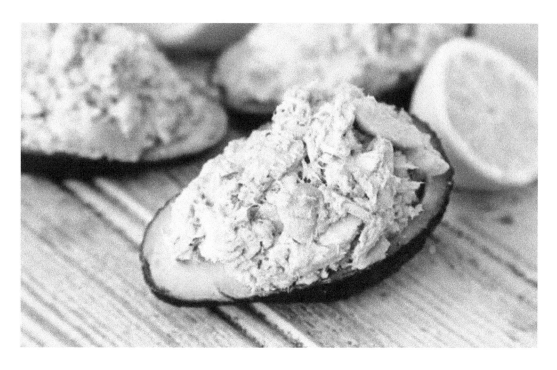

## INGREDIENTS:

(makes 2 servings)

1 extra large or 2 medium avocados, seed removed (300 g / 10.6 oz)

1 ½ cup chicken, cooked (210 g / 7.4 oz)

¼ cup mayonnaise (you can make your own) (58 g / 2 oz)

2 Tbsp sour cream or cream cheese or more mayo for dairyfree (24 g / 0.8 oz)

1 tsp thyme,

Dried 1 tsp paprika

½ tsp onion powder

½ tsp garlic powder

¼ tsp cayenne pepper

2 Tbsp fresh lemon juice

¼ tsp salt or more to taste

## DIRECTIONS:

01. Cut or shred the cooked chicken into small pieces.

02. Add the mayo, sour cream, thyme, paprika, onion powder, garlic powder, cayenne pepper...

03. Lemon juice and season with salt to taste.

04. Combine well. Scoop the middle of the avocado out leaving 1/2 - 1 inch of the avocado flesh. Cut the scooped avocado into small pieces. Place the chopped avocado into the bowl with the chicken and mix until well combined. Fill each avocado half with the chicken & avocado mixture and enjoy!

## NUTRITION:

Net carbs 5.6 g

Protein 34.5 g

Fat 50.6 g

Calories 639 kcal

Total carbs 16.6 g

Fiber 11 g

Sugars 2 g

Saturated Fat 8.6 g

Sodium 437 mg (19% RDA)

Magnesium 78 mg (19% RDA)

Potassium 1,034 mg (52% EMR)

# EGGS WITH SPINACH

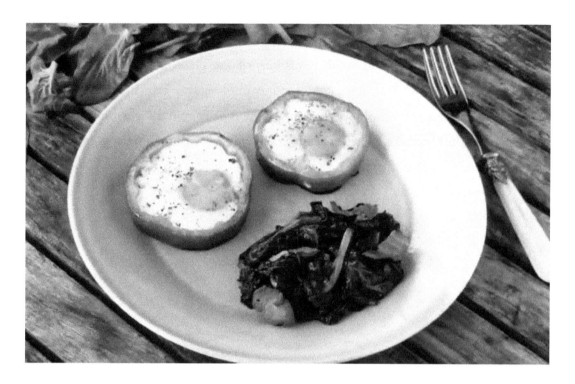

## INGREDIENTS:

2 large eggs (free range or organic)

2 rings of large green pepper, approx. 2 cm / 1 inch thick (~ 40g / 1.4 oz)

½ small red onion (30g / 1.1 oz)

1 cup fresh baby spinach (30g / 1.1 oz)

¼ cup sliced organic bacon (30g / 1.1 oz)

1 Tbsp ghee (or unsalted organic butter)

Salt and pepper to taste

Note: Try to get nitrate-free bacon or slice your own from pork belly.

## DIRECTIONS:

01. Rinse the bell pepper, remove stem and seeds. Slice it into two thick (2 cm / 1 inch) slices just near the center of the pepper (the widest part). Save the rest of the pepper for a salad or with your breakfast.

02. Grease a non-stick pan with half of the ghee or butter and add the pepper rings to

the pan. Cook on one side for about 3 minutes. Crack an egg into each of the bell pepper rings. Don't worry if some of the egg white leaks out, you can simply remove it later on with a spatula. Season with salt and ground black pepper and cook until the egg white becomes firm. When done, set aside.

03. In a separate pan, warm the remaining of the ghee or butter and add finely chopped red onion. Cook for a few minutes until slightly brown. Then, add sliced bacon and cook shortly. Add washed and drained baby spinach, season with salt and cook for another minute. Note: I already had some crispy bacon prepared in my fridge, so I just added that at the end.

04. Place everything on a serving plate and enjoy!

## NUTRITION:

Net carbs 4.3 g

Protein 17.6 g

Fat 29.3 g

Calories 360 kcal

Total carbs 6.1 g

Fiber 1.8 g

Sugars 3 g

Saturated fat 13.7 g

Sodium 575 mg (25% RDA)

Magnesium 44 mg (11% RDA)

Potassium 487 mg (24% EMR)

# KETO BREAKFAST SANDWICH

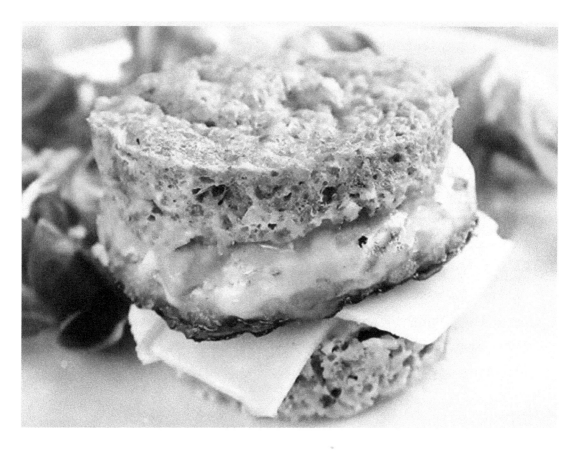

This recipe is a grain-free, healthier alternative to the popular egg McMuffin. It's vegetarian but you can add a few slices of bacon if you like. For those of you that may not have a microwave, I included some tips for baking the muffins in the oven.

## INGREDIENTS:

Muffins:

¼ cup almond flour (25 g / 0.9 oz)

¼ cup flaxmeal (38 g / 1.3 oz)

¼ tsp baking soda

1 large egg, free-range or organic

2 Tbsp heavy whipping cream or coconut milk

2 Tbsp water

¼ cup grated cheddar cheese (28 g / 1 oz)

Pinch salt

Filling:

2 large eggs, free range or organic

1 Tbsp ghee (you can make your own)

1 Tbsp butter or 2 Tbsp cream cheese for spreading

2 slices cheddar cheese or other hard type cheese (56 g / 2 oz)

1 tsp Dijon mustard (you can make your own) or 2 tsp sugar-free ketchup (you can make your own)

Salt and pepper to taste

Optional: 2 cups greens (lettuce, kale, chard, spinach, watercress, etc.) + less than 1 g net carbs per serving)

Optional: 4 slices crisped up bacon or Pancetta If you need to make this recipe nutfree, use more flaxmeal (same amount) or coconut flour (half the amount).

When using ingredients, always go by their weight, especially in case of baked goods. Measures such as cups may vary depending on a product / brand.)

## DIRECTIONS:

01. Place all the dry ingredients in a small bowl and combine well.

02. Add the egg, cream, water and mix well using a fork.

03. Grate the cheese and add it to the mixture. Combine well and place in single serving ramekins.

04. Microwave on high for 60-90 seconds. Tips for cooking in the oven: If you don't have a microwave, I suggest you make 4-8 servings at once. Preheat the oven to 175 °C/ 350 °F and cook for about 12-15 minutes or until cooked in the centre.

05. Meanwhile, fry the eggs on ghee. I used these molds to create perfect shapes for the muffin. Cook the eggs until the egg white is opaque and the yolks still runny. Season with salt and pepper and take off the heat.

06. Cut the muffins in half and spread some butter on the inside of each of the halves.

07. Top each with slices of cheese, egg and mustard. Optionally, serve with greens (lettuce, spinach, watercress, chard, etc.) and bacon.

08. Enjoy immediately! The muffins (without the filling) can be stored in an airtight container for up to 3 days.

NUTRITION:

Net carbs 3.7 g

Protein 25.6 g

Fat 54.7 g

Calories 627 kcal

Total carbs 10.2 g

Fiber 6.5 g

Sugars 1.8 g

Saturated fat 23.2 g

Sodium 638 mg (28% RDA)

Magnesium 130 mg (33% RDA)

Potassium 397 mg (20% EMR)

# INSTANT POT BEEF BOURGUIGNON

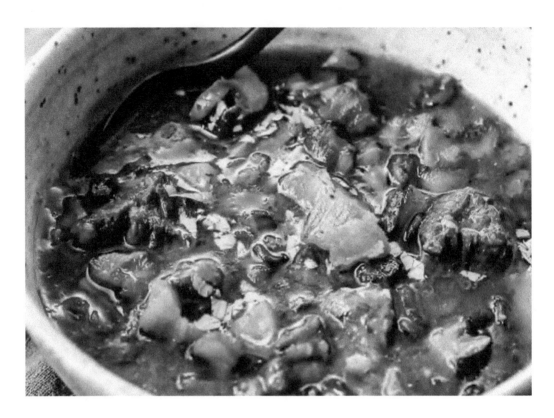

Instant Pot Beef Bourguignon is a pressure cooker recipe with beef cooked in red wine with mushrooms, onions, and carrots.

SERVINGS: 6 SERVINGS

**INGREDIENTS:**

1.5-2 lb beef chuck roast cut into ¾-inch cubes

5 strips bacon

Diced 1 small onion chopped 10 oz cremini mushrooms quartered

2 carrots chopped

5 cloves garlic minced

3 bay leaves

¾ cup dry red wine

¾ tsp xanthan gum (or corn starch, read post for directions)

1 Tbsp tomato paste

1 tsp dried thyme

Salt & pepper

## DIRECTIONS:

01. Generously season beef chunks with salt and pepper, and set aside. Select the saute mode on the pressure cooker for medium heat. When the display reads HOT, add diced bacon and cook for about 5 minutes until crispy, stirring frequently. Transfer the bacon to a paper towel lined plate.

02. Add the beef to the pot in a single layer and cook for a few minutes to brown, then flip and repeat for the other side. Transfer to a plate when done.

03. Add onions and garlic. Cook for a few minutes to soften, stirring frequently. Add red wine and tomato paste, using a wooden spoon to briefly scrape up flavorful brown bits stuck to the bottom of the pot. Stir to check that the tomato paste is dissolved. Turn off the saute mode.

04. Transfer the beef back to the pot. Add mushrooms, carrots, and thyme, stirring together. Top with bay leaves. Secure and seal the lid. Cook at high pressure for 40 minutes, followed by a manual pressure release.

05. Uncover and select the saute mode. Remove bay leaves. Evenly sprinkle xanthan gum over the pot and stir together. Let the stew boil for a minute to thicken while stirring. Turn off the saute mode. Serve into bowls and top with crispy bacon.

## NUTRITION:

Calories 673 g

Calories from Fat 288 g

Total Fat 32 g

Saturated Fat 11 g

# CRAB STUFFED MUSHROOMS

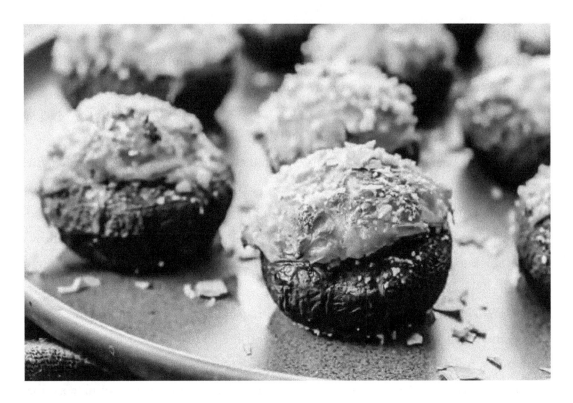

An easy recipe for crab stuffed mushrooms with cream cheese. Low carb, keto, and gluten free.

SERVINGS: 4 SERVINGS

**INGREDIENTS:**

20 oz cremini (baby bella)

Mushrooms (20-25 individual mushrooms)

2 Tbsp finely grated parmesan cheese

1 Tbsp chopped fresh parsley salt

Filling:

 4 oz cream cheese softened to room temperature

4 oz crab meat finely chopped

5 cloves garlic minced

1 tsp dried oregano

½ tsp paprika

½ tsp black pepper

¼ tsp salt

## DIRECTIONS:

01. Preheat the oven to 400 F. Prepare a baking sheet lined with parchment paper.

02. Snap stems from mushrooms, discarding the stems and placing the mushroom caps on the baking sheet 1 inch apart from each other. Season the mushroom caps with salt.

03. In a large mixing bowl, combine all filling ingredients and stir until well-mixed without any lumps of cream cheese. Stuff the mushroom caps with the mixture. Evenly sprinkle parmesan cheese on top of the stuffed mushrooms.

04. Bake at 400 F until the mushrooms are very tender and the stuffing is nicely browned on top, about 30 minutes. Top with parsley and serve while hot.

## NUTRITION:

Calories 160

Total Fat 11 g

Saturated Fat 7 g

Trans Fat 0 g

Cholesterol 58 mg

Sodium 390 mg

Potassium 300 mg

Total Carb 5.5 g

Dietary Fiber 0.5 g

Sugars 0 g

Protein 9 g

# KETO BACON CHEESEBURGER CASSEROLE

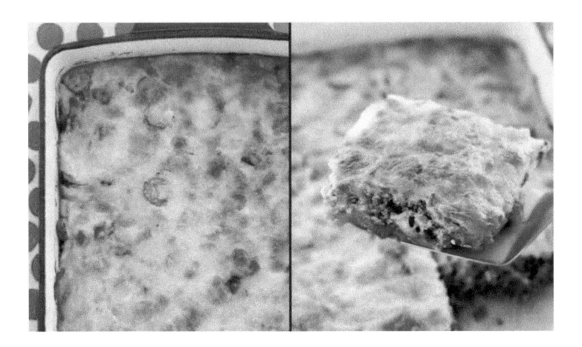

SERVINGS: 6

**INGREDIENTS:**

Beef Layer

1 onion quartered and sliced

1 clove garlic crushed

750 g ground/mince beef

60 g cream cheese full fat

3 slices bacon diced

Salt/pepper to taste

Cheats Cheese Sauce

3 eggs - medium

125 ml heavy cream

100 g shredded/grated cheese

2 Tbsp mustard

2 gherkins/pickles sliced

Salt/pepper to taste

50 g shredded/grated cheese to sprinkle over

## DIRECTIONS:

Beef Layer

01. Fry the bacon pieces until cooked then remove and set aside.

02. Fry the onion, garlic and beef until thoroughly cooked.

03. Add salt and pepper to taste, stir through the cream cheese.

04. Pour the beef layer into the baking dish. Sprinkle the bacon pieces over.

Cheats Cheese Sauce

01. Mix the eggs, cream, shredded/grated cheese, mustard, salt and pepper together. Pour the cheese sauce over the beef and bacon.

02. Place slices of gherkins/pickles all over the top then cover with the remanning shredded/grated cheese.

03. Bake at 180C/350F for 15 minutes until the cheese is golden and crispy. Serve with salad and 1 minute mayonnaise.

## NUTRITION:

Calories 613

Calories from Fat 459

Total Fat 51 g

Total Carbohydrates 3 g

Sugars 1 g

Protein 33 g

# AVOCADO COCONUT ICE CREAM

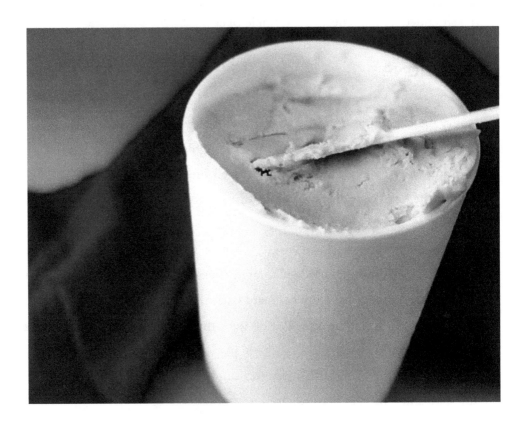

## INGREDIENTS:

1 medium avocado

1 can of coconut milk

½ cup heavy cream

¾ cup Allulose

1 medium lime

1 cup coconutflakes

## DIRECTIONS:

01. Cut avocado lengthwise and remove the pit. Scoop avocado into a blender.

02. Add coconut milk,heavycream,and sweetener into ablender with the avocado. Blend ingredients until smooth.

03. Juice and zest lime. Add lime juice and zest to blender. Blend ingredients again

for one minute. Refrigerate blended ingredients for at least one hour.

04. Preheat pan. Place coconut flakes into the pan. Toast until lightly brown around the edges. Remove pan from heat. Set aside.

05. Transfer avocado ice cream baseto the ice cream machine and churn according to manufacturer's directions.

06. Cover avocado icecreambase and freeze.

07. Serve andsprinkle with toasted coconut flakes to taste.

## NUTRITION:

Calories 222.38

Fats 21.09 g

Net Carbs 6.88 g

Protein 2.07g

# KETO CHOCOLATE MUG CAKE

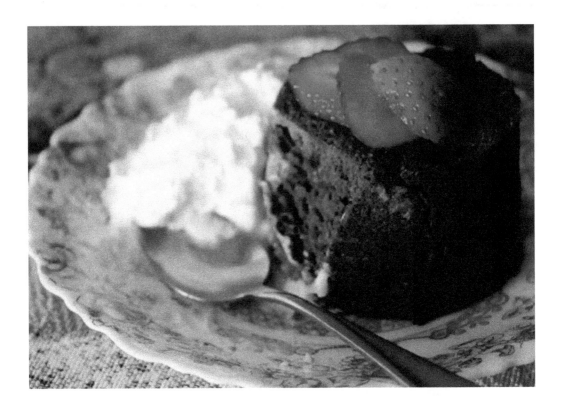

## INGREDIENTS:

2 Tbsp coconut flour

2 Tbsp unsweetenedcocoa powder

2 Tbsp Swerve confectioners

¼ tsp baking powder

2 largeeggs

2 Tbsp meltedbutter

2 Tbsp unsweetened almondmilk

## DIRECTIONS:

01. In a bowl mix together the coconut flour, unsweetened cocoa powder, Swerve confectioners,and baking powder.

02. Add the two largeeggs, melted butter, and almond milk to thedry ingredients. Mix together.

03. Add the cake batter to agreased coffee mug. You'll need onethat holds at least 12 ounces.

04. Cook the mug in the microwave for about 2 minutes. Cookingtime may varywith your microwave. Usually, Iknow it's donewhen the cakestarts puffing up overthe top of themug.

05. Remove the finished cakefrom the mug and slice in half to serve.

## NUTRITION:

Calories 219

Fats 19.06g

Net Carbs 2.95g

Protein 7.23g

# BACON AND EGG CUPS

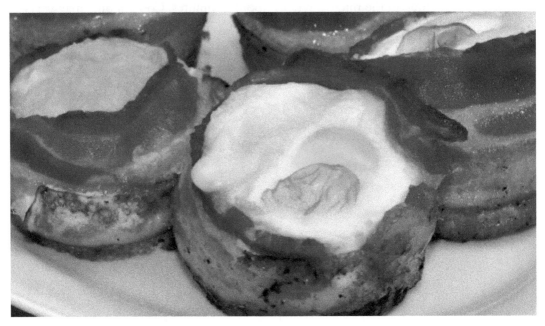

Perfect meal prep breakfast that is full of protein and portable.

SERVINGS: 12

## INGREDIENTS:

12 eggs

12 pieces nitrate free bacon (paleo approved if necessary)

1 Tbsp chopped chives salt and pepper

## NUTRITION:

Calories 67 kcal

Protein 5 g

Fat: 4 g

 Saturated Fat 1 g

Cholesterol 164 mg

Sodium 69mg

Potassium 60mg

## DIRECTIONS:

01. Preheat oven to 400 degrees.

02. Cook bacon for about 8-10 minutes. Remove from pan while still pliable, not crisp. Cool on paper towels.

03. Grease your muffin tins.

04. Put one piece of bacon in each hole, wrapping it around to line the sides. Crack the eggs in each hole. Top with chopped chives. Salt and pepper to taste.

05. Cook for about 12-15 minutes or until bacon is crisp. Watch closely.

# KETO CHOCOLATE PIE

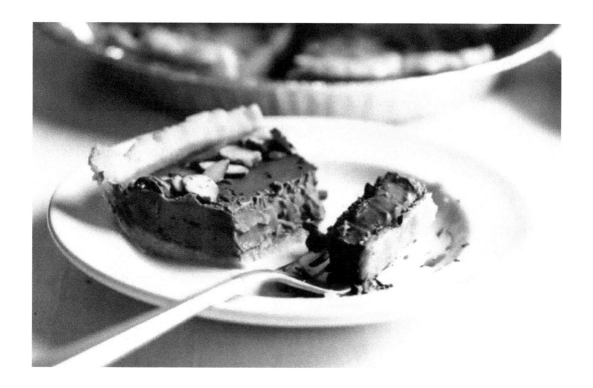

## INGREDIENTS:

2 (13.5 oz) cans chilled coconut milk, liquid discarded

½ cup almondbutter

1 tsp vanilla extract

¼ cup granulated erythritol

4 oz low-carb dark chocolate

1 cup almond flour

2 Tbsp coconut flour

2 Tbsp granulated sweetener

1 tsp xanthan gum

½ tsp sea salt

2 Tbsp ghee

1-2 Tbsp water

2 Tbsp slivered almonds, to garnish

## DIRECTIONS:

01. In a saucepan, heat the coconut cream, sweetener, vanilla, and almond butter untilthey're completely melted together.

02. Remove from heat and stir in the chocolate until the mixture is smooth and the chocolate is melted.

03. Refrigerate the mixture while you prepare the crust.

04. Whisk or sift the flours, sweetener, salt,and xanthan gum.

05. Using a fork, cut in the ghee untilthe mixture is crumbly and beginning to resemble dough.

06. Add half the water and knead into dough. If it's lookingdry, add morewater so the mixture is sticky to thetouch.

07. Press into a pie tin and bake at 350F for15 minutes or until the edgesbrown.

08. Once the crust is baked, pour the chocolate filling into the pietin andplace in the freezer for at least 4 hours.

09. Slice the pie and serve cold. Refrigerate any leftovers!

## NUTRITION:

Calories 421

Fat 41.31 g

Net Carbs 6.6g

Protein 8.7g

# KETO CREAM CHEESE BROWNIES

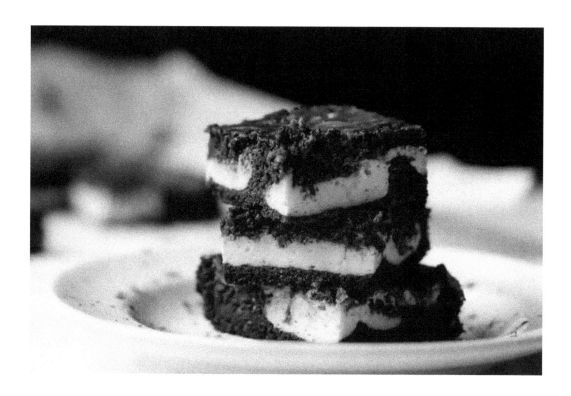

## INGREDIENTS:

For the Filling

8 oz cream cheese

¼ cup granulated erythritol

1 largeegg

For the Brownie

3 oz low carb milk chocolate

5 Tbsp butter

3 largeeggs

½ cup granulated erythritol

¼ cup cocoa powder

½ cup almondflour

## DIRECTIONS:

01. Heat oven to 350Fand line a brownie pan with parchment. Make the cheesecake filling first by beating softened cream cheese, egg for the filling, and granulated sweetener smooth. Set aside.

02. Melt the chocolate and butter at30-second intervals inthe microwave, frequently stirring until smooth. Let coolslightlywhile you prepare thebrownie.

03. Beat remaining eggs and sweetener on mediumuntil the mixture is frothy.

04. Sift in the cocoa powder and almond flour and continue to beat until thin batter forms.

05. Pour in melted chocolateand beat withthe hand mixer on low for 10 seconds. The batter will thicken to a mousse-like consistency.

06. Pour ¾ of the batter in the prepared pan, top with dollops of the cream cheese, then

Finish with the remaining brownie batter.

07. Using a spatula, smooth the batter overthe cheesecake fillingin a swirling pattern.

08. Bake for 25-30 minutes or until the center is mostly set. It may jiggle slightly but once you remove it from the oven it should firm completely. Cool before slicing!

## NUTRITION:

Calories 143.94

Fat 13.48 g

Net Carbs 1.9g

Protein 3.87g

# EASY CHEESY BACON CHICKEN

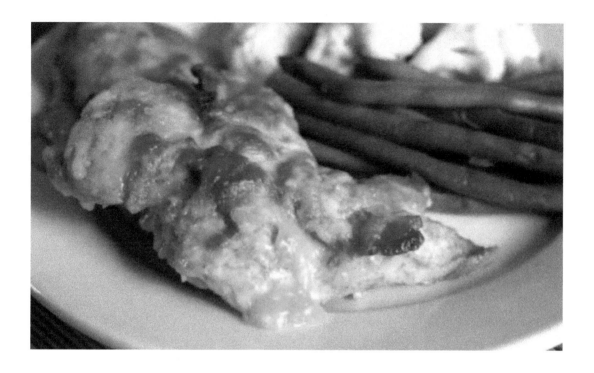

Cheesy Bacon Chicken — with only 5 ingredients: and a 5-minute preparation, you will feel the bacon love in no time!

SERVINGS: 6

## INGREDIENTS:

5-6 chicken breasts cut in half width wise (about 2.5-3 lbs.)

2 Tbsp seasoning rub (I use my smoked paprika rub, but you can use a seasoning salt or bbq rub — basically any rub with salt, garlic powder, onion powder, paprika — not an herb rub)

½ lb bacon, cut strips in half

4 oz shredded cheddar

Sugar free barbecue sauce, optional, to serve

## DIRECTIONS:

01. Preheat oven to 400. Spray a large rimmed baking sheet with cooking spray.

02. Rub both sides of chicken breasts with seasoning rub. Top each with a piece of bacon. Bake for 30 min on the top rack until the chicken is 160 degrees and the bacon looks crispy.

03. Remove tray from the oven and sprinkle the cheese oven the bacon. Put back in the oven for about 10 min until the cheese is bubbly and golden. Serve with barbecue sauce.

## NUTRITION:

Calories 345

Calories from Fat 207

Total Fat 23 g

Saturated Fat 9 g

Cholesterol 105 mg

Sodium 477 mg

Potassium 450 mg

Total Carbohydrates 1 g

Protein 29 g

# BACON & BRUSSELS SPROUT KEBABS

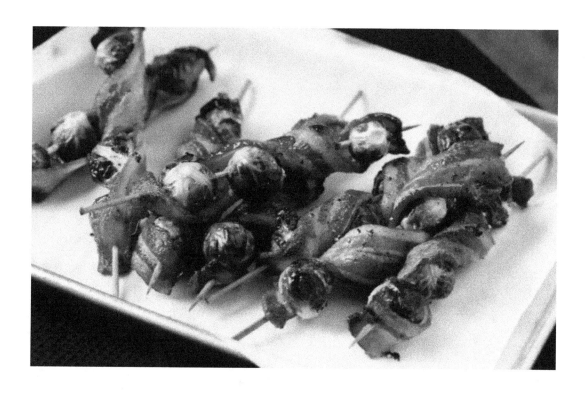

SERVINGS: 4 SERVINGS

## INGREDIENTS:

4 pieces thick cut bacon or 8 pieces of thin bacon doubled up

14 large fresh Brussels sprouts cut in half

## DIRECTIONS:

Thread the bacon and Brussels sprouts on skewers.

Bake at 400 for 35-50 minutes or until the bacon is crisp and the sprouts are tender.

## NUTRITION:

Calories 74

Total Fat 4 g

 Saturated Fat 1 g

TransFat 0 g

Cholesterol 8 mg Sugars 1 g

Sodium 152 mg Protein 5 g

Sodium 152 mg

Total Carbohydrates 6 g

Dietary Fiber 3 g

# KETO ALMOND ROLL

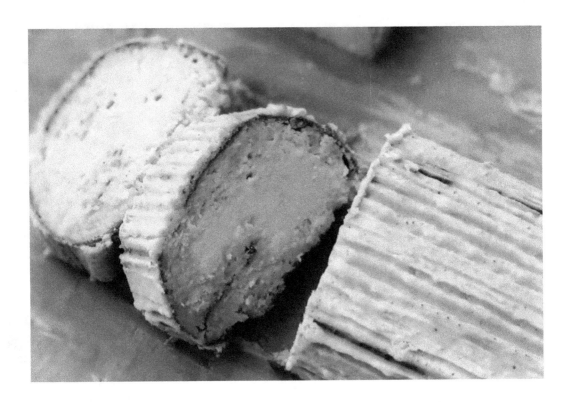

## INGREDIENTS:

For the Cake

125 g egg whites

112 g powdered erythritol/stevia blend, divided

112 g almondflour

3 g pure almond extract

For the Pumpkin Filling

260 g cream cheese softened but cool

60 g salted butter, softened

50 g powdered erythritol/stevia blend

1 tsp pure vanilla bean paste

2 tsp pumpkin spice

170 g pumpkin puree

## NUTRITION:

Calories 179.5

Fats 16.24 g

Net Carbs 3.54 g

Protein 4.76 g

## DIRECTIONS:

For the Cake

01. Preheat oven to 400F.

02. In a mixingbowl, add egg whites and 56 g sweetener.

03. Using a whisk attachment, whip to medium stiff peaks.Stop when themeringue holds its shape.

04. In a separate bowl, combine the remaining 56 g sweetener, almond flour, and flavoring.

05. Whisk to combineuntil homogenous.

06. In three additions, gentlyfold in the dry mixture into the egg whites. Use the biggestrubber spatula you have, thisensures less frequentfoldingthus keeping the air in the sponge intact.

07. Evenly spread thebatteron a grease and parchment (or baking foil) lined quarter sheet tray, approx 9" X 13" jelly roll pan.

08. Bake for 10-12 minutes. Invert onto a parchment lined wire rack to cool.


For the Pumpkin Filling

01. In a medium bowl, beat the cream cheese until smooth.

02. Add the sweetener. Continue until fluffyand light.

03. Add vanillapaste and pumpkin spice. Beat until well incorporated.

04. In two intervals, add the pumpkin puree, scraping the bowl in between addition.

05. Add the butter and beat until themixture comes together. Your filling should be smooth and light. Adjust the sweetness with more some liquid stevia, to taste.

06. Refrigerate until ready to use. Make sure to re-whip (by hand is fine) until fluffy before using.


Assembly

01. Evenly spread thefilling over thesponge.

02. Gently rollto form into alog, using the parchment to lift the cake. I find that rolling the cake from the shorter side yields a thicker roll and less cracking. Refrigerate untilready to serve.

# RASPBERRY ICE CREAM

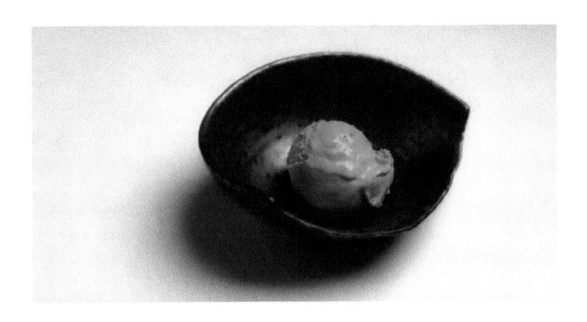

## INGREDIENTS:

680 g (24 oz) raspberries frozen

150 g (5 oz) allulose

50 g (2 oz) fromage blanc

225 g (8 oz) heavy whipping cream

## NUTRITION:

Calories 73.16

Fats 5.42 g

Net Carbs 4.04g

Protein 1.12g

## DIRECTIONS:

01. Place frozen raspberries in a bowl. Leave to thaw at room temperature about 30 minutes to an hour.

02. Meanwhile, in a separatebowl, mix to combinethe fromage blanc and heavywhipping cream.Refrigerate.

03. When the raspberries have thawed and softened, place in a blender and puree. Pass through a fine-meshed strainer and discard seeds.

04. Stirin allulose. Mix until dissolved.

05. Pour raspberry mixture onto thecreammixture. Mix until homogeneous. Refrigerate for at least 4 hours.

06. Using an ice cream maker, churnper manufacturers directions.

# KETO CHOCOLATE DONUTS

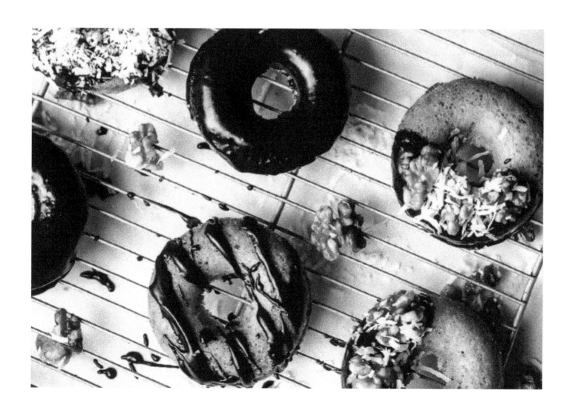

**INGREDIENTS:**

Donut

2 Tbsp butter softened

½ cup erythritol

2 largeeggs

¼ cup unsweetened almond milk

1 tsp vanilla

1 cup almond flour

1 Tbsp psyllium husk powder

1 Tbsp bakingpowder

Chocolate Coating

2 oz unsweetened baker's chocolate

3 Tbsp butter

2 Tbsp powdered erythritol

Toffee Nuts

⅓ cup raw walnuts

1 Tbsp erythritol

½ Tbsp butter Pinch of sea salt

1 Tbsp unsweetenedcoconut, optional garnish

## DIRECTIONS:

Donut

01. Heat oven to 350Fand prepare a6 welled donut pan with non-stick cooking spray. Cream the softened butter and sugar together until the butter and sugar are evenly mixed.

02. Add two eggs and beat with a hand mixer or whisk until the eggs are light and frothy.

03. Pour in milk and vanilla and beatagain just to make sure all of the ingredients are mixed well.

04. Using a sifter or mesh colander, add halfof the dry ingredients to the wet andmix well.

05. Finish by sifting the remaining dry ingredients and stir until batter forms.

06. Pour batter into prepared donut pan and bake for 20 minutes or until the donuts begin to brown.Cool completely before removing from pan.

Chocolate Coating

07. Melt unsweetened chocolate and butterin a microwave-safe dish. Mix in powdered Erythritol and set aside until the donuts are ready for dipping.

Toffee Nut Topping

08. Heat nuts, sweetener, and butter in a small microwave-safe dish for 45 seconds at a time, stirringfrequently until the nuts begin to caramelize.

09. Spread nuts on parchment paperand sprinkle with salt.

10. Dip the donuts inthe liquid chocolate or drizzleover the top.

11. Top with toffee nuts andoptional shredded coconut. Store in an airtight container.

NUTRITION:

Calories 340.83

Fat 31.11 g

Net Carbs 4.81g

Protein 8.64g

# KETO FLAN

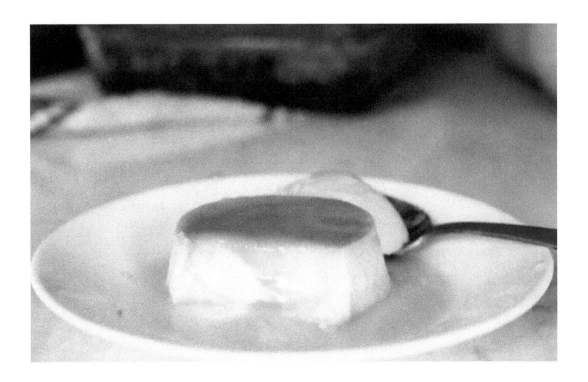

## INGREDIENTS:

⅓ Cup erythritol, for caramel

⅛ Cup water

1 Tbsp butter

1 cup heavy whipping cream

2 largeeggs

2 large egg yolks

1 Tbsp vanilla

¼ cup erythritol, forcustard

## DIRECTIONS:

01. In a deep pan, heat up the erythritol forthe caramel. Stir it frequently.

02. Add the water and butter.

03. Stiroccasionally until the sauce has become a golden brown.

04. Pour into the bottom of each ramekin, covering the bottom nicely. Set aside and let them cool.

05. In abowl, mix together the heavywhipping cream, remaining erythritol, and vanilla.

06. In a separate bowl, whisktogether your whole eggs. Then add in the yolks, whisking once more.

07. Slowly stir your eggs into the cream mix.

08. Pour the custard into each ramekin, on top of the caramel.

09. Place the ramekins into a casserole dish and fill over halfway with hot water. Bake at350F for 30 minutes. Take the casserole dish out of the oven butleave the ramekins in the hotwater for another 10minutes.

10. Using tongs take out theramekins and let them sit forat least 4 hours, or overnight, in the fridge.

11. When ready to eat, take a knife and slowly run it on the insideof the custard to release it from the ramekin.

12. Turn the ramekin upside down and slowly jiggle the custard onto the plate.

13. Enjoy!

## NUTRITION:

Calories 298

Fats 31.5g

Net Carbs 2.4 g

Protein 4.5 g

# BACON SPINACH DIP

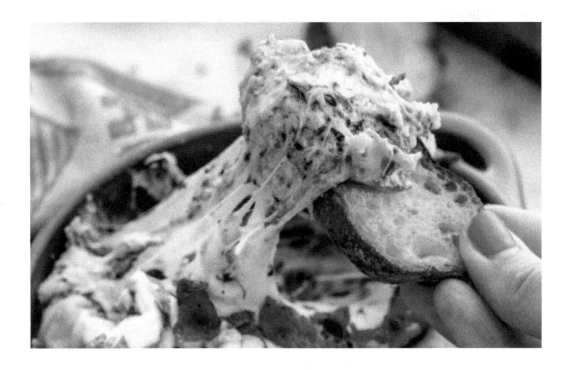

This is the ultimate spinach dip recipe! I've eaten spinach dip so very many times in my life but this one beats them all. It is cheesy, creamy, garlicky, and perfect with fresh veggies or crackers.

SERVINGS: 8

## INGREDIENTS:

12 oz bacon cooked until crisp and crumbled

4 oz cream cheese

¼ cup mayo

¼ cup sour cream

1 tsp garlic powder

½ cup grated parmesan cheese

16 oz frozen spinach thawed and drained well

6 oz shredded mozzarella

## DIRECTIONS:

01. Preheat oven to 350.

02. Cook bacon until crisp, drain, and crumbled or chop it into small pieces.

03. In a large bowl mix the cream cheese, mayo, garlic powder, and parmesan cheese. Mix in the spinach, half the bacon, and half the mozzarella.

04. Spread in a deep dish pie plate. Sprinkle the remaining mozzarella and bacon on top.

05. Bake at 350 until hot and bubbly. About 15 minutes.

NOTES: Alternatively, you can microwave the dip for about 5 minutes. The only down side to microwaving is the cheese doesn't get golden on top. But on a hot summer day that is a sacrifice I am willing to make. Also, if you are an artichoke fan feel free to add some for a Bacon Caesar Spinach Artichoke Dip.

## NUTRITION:

Calories 395

Calories from Fat 315

Total Fat 35 g

Saturated Fat 13 g

Cholesterol 72 mg

Sodium 648 mg

Potassium 338 mg

Total Carbohydrates 4 g

Dietary Fiber 1 g

Sugars 1 g

Protein 15 g

# CHEDDAR CHICKEN BREASTS

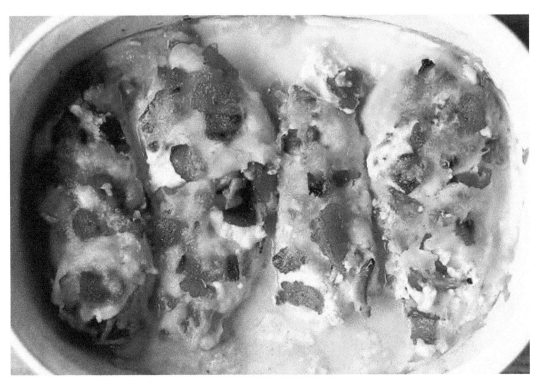

Looking for easy baked chicken recipes? Do you like chicken and cream cheese together? Then, this Bacon, Cream Cheese, and Cheddar Chicken is a great choice! Super easy to make! And, you use simple ingredients. This chicken bake is low carb, high fat, KETO friendly, gluten free recipe.

SERVINGS: 4 SERVINGS

**INGREDIENTS:**

1 Tbsp olive oil

4 chicken breasts (use 4 thin chicken breasts, or use 2 large chicken breasts, sliced in half, horizontally)

Salt and pepper

6 oz cream cheese, cold, refrigerated, and sliced into 8 slices

8 strips bacon, cooked, chopped

1 cup Cheddar cheese, shredded

## DIRECTIONS:

01. Preheat the oven to 400 F.

02. Grease the bottom of the casserole dish with olive oil. I used the the oval casserole dish measured 13 inches x 9 inches x 4 inches deep.

03. Add chicken breasts to the casserole dish. Note about chicken: use 4 thin chicken breasts, or use 2 large thick chicken breasts, sliced in half horizontally each to make 4 thin chicken breasts. 04. Sprinkle chicken breasts with salt and pepper.

05. Top with cream cheese. Cream cheese should be cold, right out of the fridge, sliced into 8 thin slices.

06. Top with chopped cooked bacon (drained from fat).

07. Top with shredded Cheddar cheese.

08. Bake, uncovered, for about 20-30 minutes, until the chicken is cooked through. The cooking time will depend on the thickness of your chicken breasts.

## NUTRITION:

Calories 602

Calories from Fat 423

Total Fat 47 g

Saturated Fat 21 g

Cholesterol 177 mg

Sodium 734 mg

Potassium 591 mg

Total Carbohydrates 2 g

Sugars 1 g

Protein 39 g

# KETO BACON MAC 'N' CHEESE

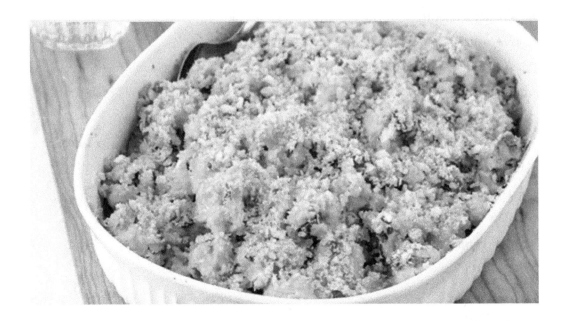

This is a fabulous meal for those of you following a low-carb diet or anyone just craving some good old-fashioned comfort food.

## INGREDIENTS:

Coconut oil, for the dish

1 large head cauliflower (about 1 & ⅔ pounds / 750 g), cored and broken into ½-inch (1.25-cm) pieces

⅓ Cup finely chopped fresh parsley (22 g)

6 strips bacon (about 6 oz/170 g), cooked until crisp, then crumbled (reserve the grease)

2 cups unsweetened non-dairy milk (475 ml)

2 Tbsp unflavored gelatin

1 Tbsp fresh lemon juice

1 tsp onion powder

1 tsp finely ground gray sea salt

¼ tsp garlic powder

⅓ Cup

## NUTRITION:

al yeast (22 g)

2 large eggs, beaten

 2 tsp prepared yellow mustard

2 oz pork dust or ground pork rinds (60 g)

## DIRECTIONS:

01. Preheat the oven to 350°F (177°C) and grease a shallow 1½-quart (1.4-L) casserole dish with coconut oil. Set aside.

02. Place the cauliflower, parsley, and bacon in a large bowl and toss to combine.

03. Place the reserved bacon grease, milk, gelatin, lemon juice, onion powder, salt, and garlic powder in a medium-sized saucepan. Bring to a boil over medium heat, whisking occasionally. Once boiling, continue to boil for 5 minutes.

04. Whisk in the nutrition al yeast, eggs, and mustard and gently cook for 3 minutes, whisking constantly.

05. Remove the saucepan from the heat and pour the "cheese" sauce over the cauliflower mixture. (If you've overcooked the sauce or didn't whisk it well enough, you may end up with small pieces of cooked egg; for an ultra-smooth sauce, pour the sauce through a fine-mesh strainer.) Toss with a spatula until all the cauliflower pieces are coated in the cheese sauce.

06. Transfer the coated cauliflower to the prepared casserole dish and smooth it out with the back of a spatula. Sprinkle the pork dust evenly over the top. Bake for 40 to 45 minutes, until the cauliflower is fork-tender, checking with a sharp knife on the edge of the casserole.

07. Allow to sit for 15 minutes before serving.

08. STORE IT: Keep in an airtight container in the fridge for up to 3 days.

09. REHEAT IT: Microwave until the desired temperature is reached. Or place in a covered casserole dish and reheat in a preheated 300°F (150°C) oven for 10 to 15 minutes, until warmed through. Or reheat in a frying pan, covered, on medium-low.

10. PREP AHEAD: Prepare the cheese sauce up to 2 days in advance. Bring it to a light simmer before continuing with Step 5.

11. SERVE IT WITH: Add a dollop or two of mayonnaise.

NUTRITION: (per serving)

Calories 440

Calories from fat 244

Total fat 27 g

Saturated fat 8.8 g

Cholesterol 128 mg

Sodium 973 mg

Carbs 14.6 g

Dietary fiber 6.6 g

Net carbs 8 g

Sugars 4.8 g

Protein 34.6 g

# KETO CHOCOLATE CAKE

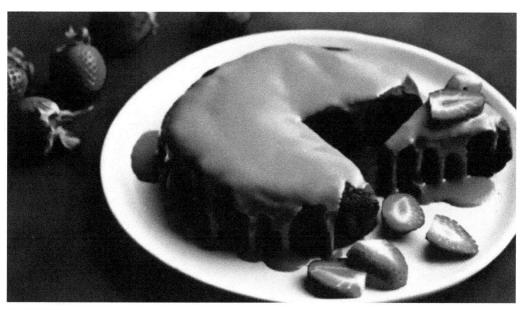

SERVES: 8

INGREDIENTS:

Chocolate Cake

½ cupcoconut flour

5 eggs separated

½ cup coconut oil or grass-fed ghee,melted

½ cup coconut cream

2 tsp vanilla extract or 1 tsp vanilla powder

4 Tbsp granulated sweetener(or more to taste), such as birch xylitol, nonGMO erythritol, or MitoSweet

½ cup cacao powder

Pinch of salt

Additional grass-fed butter, ghee, or coconut oil forgreasing


Chocolate Glaze

1 cup coconut cream

1 Tbsp ghee or coconut oil

1 tsp vanilla extract

1 Tbsp cacao powder

1 Tbsp erythritol, xylitol, or MitoSweet, or roughly 10 drops of liquid stevia

Pinch of salt

## DIRECTIONS:

01. Preheat oven to 350 degrees. Grease an8-inch metal cake panwith butter, ghee, or coconut oil.

02. Whisk eggwhitesuntil they develop a foamy consistency.

03. In a separate bowl, mix all remaining chocolate cake ingredients. Then slowly fold egg whites into the batter.

04. Pour batter into cake pan. Bake for 25 minutes, or untila knife inserted into the center of the cake comes out clean.

05. While ketochocolate cake cools, prepare glaze. In a saucepan on low heat, add all glaze ingredients and whiskcontinuously to combine.

06. Pour chocolate glaze intoa glass jar and drizzle over the cake. Serve keto chocolate cake warm, or store covered on your counter or in the refrigerator (icing will harden).

## NUTRITION:

Calories 321

Total Fat 30 g

Sodium 65 mg

Total Carbs 22.4 g

DietaryFiber 5.5 g

TotalSugars 1.9 g

Sugaralcohols 12 g

Net Carbs 4.9g

Protein 6.5 g

Potassium 158 mg

Cholesterol 106 mg

Vitamin D 10 mcg

Iron 2mg

Calcium 27 mg

# KETO CAKE WITH CHOCOLATE AVOCADO FROSTING

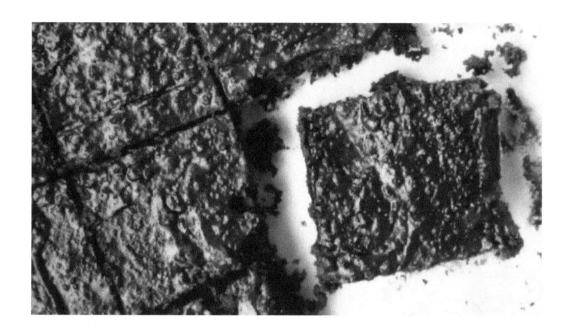

SERVES: 12

## INGREDIENTS:

Sheet Cake

½ cup coconut oil melted

½ cup cold-brewed coffee

3 Tbsp cacao powder

½ tsp cinnamon

1 cup almond flour

½ cup coconut flour

1 tsp baking soda

¼ cup liquid monk fruit extract

1 tsp vanilla extract "Buttermilk" (½ cup almond milk + 1 ½ Tbsp apple cider vinegar)

2 eggs

Chocolate Avocado Frosting

½ large avocado (about 3 Tbsp)

2 Tbsp cacao powder

1 Tbsp coconut oil

¼ cup unsweetened lite coconut milk (or dilute 1/8cup full-fat coconut milk with1/8 cup water)

2 tsp liquid monk fruit extract

## DIRECTIONS:

01. Preheat the oven to 400 degrees.

02. In a small mixing bowl, combine coconutoil, cold brew, cacao powder,and cinnamon.

03. In a large mixing bowl, combine the almond flour, coconut flour, baking soda,and monk fruit extract.

04. In the small mixing bowl, whisk togetherthe "buttermilk" (almond milk + apple cider vinegar), eggs,and vanilla extract, then add to the mixturein the large mixing bowl.

05. Mix everything until completely combined. You may use an electric mixer, but this works just as well mixing by hand.

06. Add the batter toa 9×13bakingdish and bake for 20 minutes.

07. Once finished, remove from the oven and allowcooling while you make the frosting.

08. Combine all frosting ingredients together and mix witha mixer, blender/ food processor, or by hand until completely smooth.

09. Once the cake is completely cooled, spread the frosting, then cut into slices.

## NUTRITION:

Calories 208

Protein 4 g

Carbohydrates 8 g

Fiber 4 g

Net Carbs 4 g

Sugar <1 g Iron 9g

Fat 18 g Calcium 7 g

Saturated Fat 10 g Potassium 98 g

Unsaturated Fat 8 g. Cholesterol 31 g

# GLUTEN-FREE CHOCOLATE COCONUT CUPCAKES

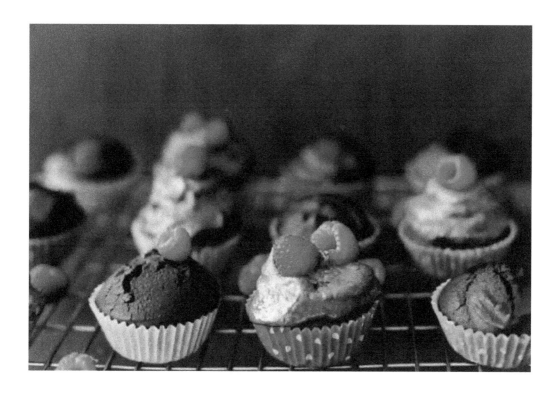

MAKES: 20 CUPCAKES

## INGREDIENTS:

Cupcakes: 1 cup coconut flour sifted

250g grass-fedbutter or ghee

Pinch of salt

7 large eggs or 8 small-medium sized eggs

½ cup cacao butter

½ cup cocoa powder

½ tsp baking soda

½ tsp paleo baking powder

1 tsp apple cider vinegar

2 tsp vanilla powder

2 tsp cinnamon

1 cup of xylitolor sweetener of choice

Icing:

¼ cup cacao butter

¼ cocoa powder

Pinch of salt

2-3 Tbsp Brain Octane Oil

⅓ cup coconut cream Xylitolor sweetener of choice

Garnish: Fresh berries

**NUTRITION:**

Calories 183

Total fat 21.6 g

Sat Fat 11 g

Cholesterol 92mg

Sodium 73.5 mg

Total Carb 5.7g

Dietary Fiber 3.8 g

Sugars 1.4 g

Protein 4 g

## DIRECTIONS:

01. Preheat the oven to 350°F (170°C). Line two trays of muffin tins with paper cups.

02. Add the cacao powder and butter to a small saucepan and heat over low to mediumheat until completely melted and incorporated.

03. Add all ingredients to a food processor and blend until smoothand creamy.

04. Taste the mixture and adjust if needed; adding a touchof extra sweetener ofyour choice, cinnamon, vanilla, or a little more salt to enhance the chocolate flavor.

05. Spoon the mixture into the prepreparedmuffin trays evenly.

06. Place in the oven and bake for roughly 20 minutes.

07. While the cupcakes bake, add allthe icing ingredients to a small saucepan and melt on a low to medium heat until completely combined.

08. Taste the icing mixture and adjust the sweetness if needed. Pour into a bowl,then place in the fridge to set.

09. When the muffinsare golden brown and cooked through, remove them fromthe oven and let them cool.

10. Remove the chilled icing from the fridge. As an optional step, scoop the icingout and

re-blend to create a lighter and fluffier icing. Spread over the tops of the cooled muffinsand garnishwith berries.

11. Store in the fridge.

# KETO RASPBERRY STUFFED CAKE

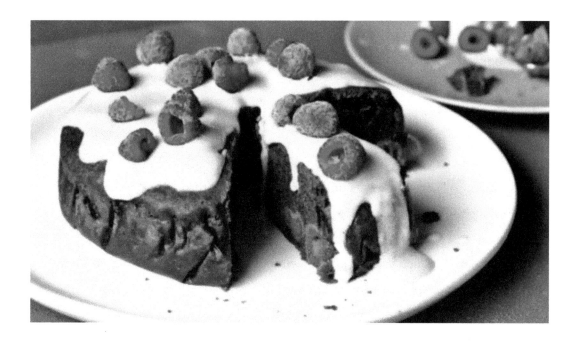

SERVES: 8

**INGREDIENTS:**

Cake:

5 oz cacao butter melted

2 oz grass-fed ghee

½ cup coconutcream

1 cup green banana flour

3 tsp pure vanilla extract or 2tsp vanilla powder

4 eggs

½ cup your choice granulated sweetener, such as Lakanto MonkFruit

1 tsp baking powder

2 tsp apple cider vinegar

2 cup raspberries

White chocolate sauce:

3 ½ oz cacao butter

½ cup coconut cream

2 tsp pure vanilla extract

Pinch of salt

## DIRECTIONS:

For cake

01. Preheat oven to 280 degrees.

02. Combine all dry ingredients untilthoroughly mixed through.

03. Leaving the raspberries aside, add all ofthe remainingingredients and mix until well combined.

04. Line a small, 8-inch cake or loaf tin withbakingpaper,and pour in the cake mix.

05. Scatter the raspberries (reserving somefor garnishing) over the top of the cake mix.As the cake bakes, they will sink towards the bottom of the cake.

06. Place in your oven and bake for1 hour,or until firm.

07. While it bakes, prepare the sauce.

For sauce:

01. Combine all ingredients in a saucepan on low heat.

02. Use a fork to mixall ingredientswell toensurethe cacao butter combines with the cream.

03. Remove from theheat and set aside to cool to room temperature. If it's too cool, it will harden, and ifit is too warm, it willbe slightly runny.

04. Drizzle on each individualpiece of cake when serving, or drizzle over the top of the entire cake ifthis iswhat you prefer.

05. Scatter the cake with extra raspberries,and serve.

## NUTRITION:

| | | | |
|---|---|---|---|
| Calories 323 | Carbohydrates 9.8 g | Protein 4 g | Calcium 25 mg |
| TotalFat 31.5 g | Dietary Fiber 3.2g | Cholesterol 82 mg | Iron 1mg |
| Sodium 55mg | Net Carbs 6.6 g | Potassium 223 mg | |
| | Total Sugars 4.8 g | Vitamin D 8 mcg | |

# LOW-CARB BANANA PUDDING

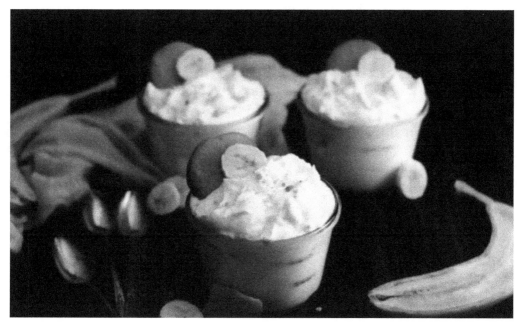

SERVES: 6

## INGREDIENTS:

Vanilla Wafer

¾ cup almondflour

⅓ cup granulated stevia erythritol blend

1/8 tsp bakingsoda

1/8 tsp salt

4 Tbsp almond milk

1 egg, separated

2 tsp vanilla extract


Banana Pudding

⅓ cupgranulated stevia erythritol plus blend, separated 3 Tbsp

1 tsp xanthamgum

Pinch of salt

3 egg yolks

1 tsp vanilla extract

¼ tsp natural banana flavor (optional)

1 ½ cup organic grass-fed heavy cream

¼ of a banana, thinly sliced

## DIRECTIONS:

Vanilla wafer

01. Preheat oven to 375 degrees Fahrenheit. Line 2cookiesheetswith parchment paper.

02. In a medium bowl, combine almond flour, sweetener baking soda, and salt. Gradually add 4 tablespoons milk, stirring between each addition.

03. Whisk in egg yolk and vanilla extract until smooth.

04. Place egg white in a small bowl. Using ahand mixer beat egg white until stiffpeaks form.

05. Gently fold half ofthe whipped egg white into the almond flour mixture to lighten, then fold in the remainder of the egg white being careful notbreak down the fluffiness.

06. Transfer batter toa pastry bag with a small circular tip.Pipe 1"-1 1/2"circular wafers leavingat least 1 ½ inches between each wafer. Alternatively, you can simply place by teaspoonfuls onto thebakingsheets.You will end up with about 18 mounds of dough.

07. Place in oven andbake for 15-17minutes or until golden brown.

08. When finished baking, remove from oven. Let cool about 5 minutes on the baking sheet, then transfer to a cooling rack usinga spatula andlet cool to room temperature.

Banana Pudding Directions

01. In a medium saucepan, whisk together sweetener, xanthin gum and salt. Addthe yolks, and stir until combined.

02. Gradually add 1 ½ cup cream, stirring until smooth between each addition. Mixture should begin thicken.

03. Place saucepan over medium low heat, stirring constantly. Heat for 3-4 minutes or until mixture begins to boil.

04. Remove pudding from heat and let cool to room temperature.Stir in 1 teaspoon

vanilla extractand banana flavor, if using.

05. Ina medium bowl, beat1 cup heavy cream with an electric blender until stiff peaksform. Add 3tbsp sweetener and ½ tsp vanilla and beat just untilcombined.

06. Add the whippedcreaminto the cooled pudding, folding to combine.

To serve

01. Layer pudding, banana slices andwafersas desired.

## NUTRITION:

Calories 335

Fat 30.2 g

Carbs 5.5 g

Fiber 2 g

Protein 5.5 g

Net carbs 3.5g

# RASPBERRY LEMON POPSICLES

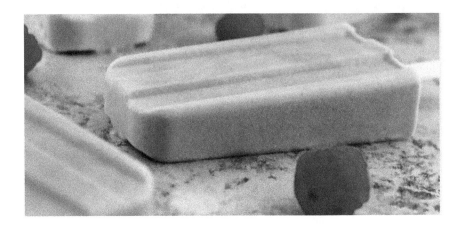

## INGREDIENTS:

100 g Raspberries Juice

½ Lemon

¼ cup Coconut Oil

1 cup Coconut Milk

¼ cup Sour Cream

¼ cup Heavy Cream

½ tsp Guar Gum

20 drops Liquid Stevia

## NUTRITION:

Calories 151

Fats 16g

NetCarbs 2 g

Protein 0.5 g

## DIRECTIONS:

01. Add all ingredients into a container and use an immersion blender to blend the mixture together.

02. Continue blendinguntil the raspberries are completely mixed in with the restof the ingredients.

03. Strain the mixture, making sure to discard all raspberryseeds.

04. Pour the mixture into molds. I use this mold formy popsicles. Set the popsicles in the freezer for a minimum of 2 hours.

05. Run the mold under hot water todislodge the popsicles.

06. Serve andeat whenever you want!

# GLUTEN-FREE SPICED KETO COOKIES

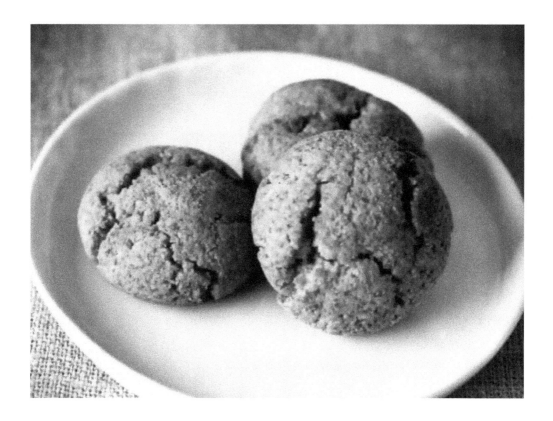

SERVINGS: 18

**INGREDIENTS:**

Cream Together

4 Tbsp softened butter or coconut oil

2 Tbsp agavenectar

1 egg

2 Tbsp water

Add Dry ingredients

2.5 cup Almond Flour

½ cup sugar

2 tsp ground ginger

1 tsp ground cinnamon

½ tsp Ground Nutmeg

1 tsp BakingSoda ¼ tsp Salt

## DIRECTIONS:

01. Preheat the oven to 350F.

02. Line a cookie sheet with parchment paper and set aside.

03. Using a hand blender, cream together the butter, agave nectar, egg, and water.

04. To this mixture, add all the dry ingredients and mix well on low speed.

05. Roll into 2tsp balls and arrange on a baking tray with parchment paper. Theydon't really spreadtoo much but leave a little room between them.

06. Bake for 12-15 mins untilthe tops have lightly browned.

07. Once cooled, store in an air-tightcontainer. Forlike, the one hour these will be around beforeyou eat them all.

## NUTRITION:

Calories 122 kcal

Fat 10g

Saturated fat 2 g

Carbohydrates 5 g

Fiber 1g

Sugar 2 g

Protein 3 g

# CHOCOLATE CHIP KETO COOKIES

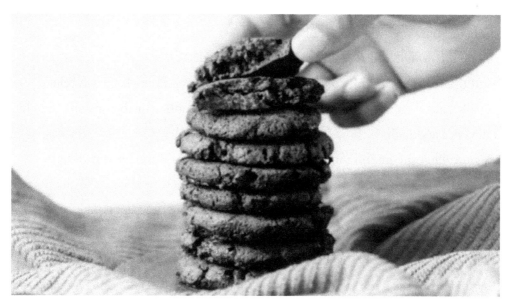

MAKES: 10

## INGREDIENTS:

2 cups blanched organic almond meal

¼ cup grass-fed butter or ghee, melted

2 Tbsp Collagen Powder (or 1Tbsp Collagelatin)

¼ cup cocoa powder

½–¾ cup Lakanto (or sweetener of choice)

1 tsp vanilla

1 egg

½ tsp paleo baking powder

1 tsp apple cider vinegar

2 tsp cinnamon (optional)

A pinch of salt

⅓ cup Chocolate FuelBar, orother high-quality dark chocolate, chopped

## DIRECTIONS:

01. Preheat the oven to 350F. Grease and line a baking tray with parchment paper.

02. Add all your ingredients to a food processor except thechocolate chips and collagen,and blitz to combine evenly.

03. Taste the dough and adjust the sweetness if needed.

04. Add the collagen and blend gently to avoid destroying the delicate protein.

05. Finally, add the chocolatechips and givethe mix a gentle stir to combine the chips into the cookie dough.

06. Begin rolling the mixture into balls and place them onto the lined baking tray.

07. Press the balls as flat as you like, they won't rise much,so if you like them softer andmore chewykeep them quite full. However if youlike a crunchier cookie, pressthem flat intoeven well-formed cookies.

08. Place the cookies in the oven and bake for 10-12 minutes, or until golden brown.

09. Remove from the oven when they're ready andplace the cookies onto a wirecooling rack.

10. Enjoy witha hot mug of bulletproof coffee.

11. Store the leftovers in an airtightcontainer when they're completely cooled.

## NUTRITION:

Calories 287

TotalFat 16.5 g

Sodium 154 mg

Carbohydrates 6.5 g

Dietary Fiber 4 g

TotalSugars 0.8 g

Protein 6.5 g

Potassium 280 mg

Magnesium 333 mg

# KETO BACONWRAPPED JALAPENO POPPERS

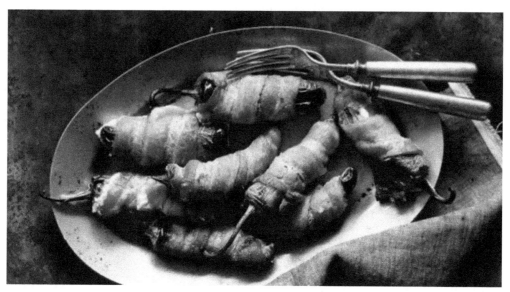

Cheddar and cream cheese gets stuffed into jalapenos and then wrapped in bacon and baked until the cheese is gooey and the bacon is crispy!

SERVINGS: 8

## INGREDIENTS:

8 large-ish jalapeno peppers

3 oz (85 g) sharp yellow cheddar, shredded

3 oz (85 g) full-fat cream cheese

8 slices bacon Avocado oil spray

## DIRECTIONS:

01. Preheat the oven to 400F.

02. Cut a thin slit down the length of each pepper and carefully remove the inner ribs and seeds, trying to keep the pepper itself as intact as possible.

03. Use a fork to mash together the cheddar and cream cheeses in a small bowl.

04. Stuff the cheese mixture into each pepper, closing each pepper up as much as possible.

05. Wrap a slice of bacon around the outside of each pepper, securing with a toothpick if necessary.

06. Lightly spray each popper with avocado oil.

07. Arrange the poppers on a large baking sheet and bake until the bacon is crispy, about 20 minutes. You can broil the poppers for a couple minutes at the end if you want to brown them more.

08. Serve.

## NUTRITION:

Calories 131

Fat 10.2 g

Potassium 174 g

Net Carbs 2.7 g

Carbohydrates 4 g

Sodium 239 g

Fiber 1.3 g

Protein 6.2 g

# KETO DEVILED EGGS RECIPE WITH AVOCADO AND BACON

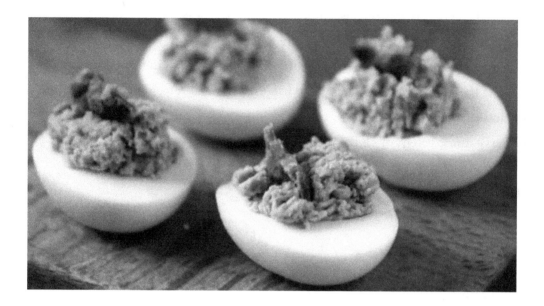

Mexican deviled eggs make a delicious and simple deviled egg recipe! These naturally keto deviled eggs with avocado and bacon are easy to make, with common ingredients. Such a flavorful take on avocado deviled eggs!

SERVINGS: 6

## INGREDIENTS:

6 large Egg

2 Tbsp Avocado (just scoop with a measuring spoon)

2 Tbsp Mayonnaise

1 tsp Lime juice

¾ tsp Taco seasoning (use salted seasoning; add ¼ tsp salt if seasoning is unsalted)

½ cup Tomatoes (finely chopped, seeds removed and liquid drained; divided)

¼ cup Bacon bits (cooked; divided)

2 tsp Fresh cilantro (chopped)

1 pinch Cayenne pepper (optional — to taste)

## DIRECTIONS:

01. Boil eggs for 8-9 minutes according to the directions here.

02. Peel the eggs and cut them in half. Take out the yolks and place them into a bowl.

03. Add the avocado, mayonnaise, lime juice, and taco seasoning to the yolks.
Mash until smooth. If desired, add cayenne pepper to taste.

04. Fold in half of the tomatoes and half of the bacon bits to the yolk mixture.

05. Stuff the mixture into the egg white halves. Top with remaining tomatoes, bacon bits, and cilantro.

06. Serve immediately, or chill until ready to serve.

## NUTRITION:

Calories 134

Fat 10 g

Protein 7 g

Total Carbs 1 g

Net Carbs 1 g

Fiber 0 g

# AVOCADO & EGG FAT BOMBS

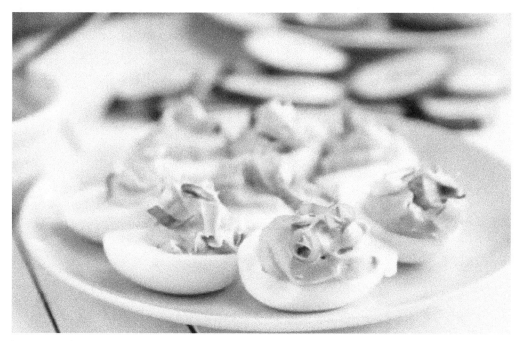

SERVINGS: 5

## INGREDIENTS:

3 large cooked egg yolks

½ large avocado, peeled and seed removed (100 g/ 3.5 oz)

¼ cup mayonnaise (55 g/ 1.9 oz) - you can make your own

1 Tbsp lemon or lime juice

½ tsp salt, or to taste freshly ground black pepper

2 Tbsp chopped spring onions or chives

## DIRECTIONS:

01. Start by cooking the eggs. Fill a small saucepan with water up to three quarters. Add a good pinch of salt. This will prevent the eggs from cracking. Bring to a boil. Using a spoon or hand, dip each egg in and out of the boiling water — be careful not to get burnt. This will prevent the egg from cracking as the temperature change won't be so sudden. To get the eggs hard-boiled, you need round 10 minutes. This timing works for large eggs. When done, remove from the heat and place in a bowl filled with

cold water. I like and always use this egg timer! When the eggs are chilled, peel off the shells.

02. Halve the avocado and remove the seed and peel. Cut the eggs in half and carefully — without breaking the egg whites — spoon the egg yolks into a bowl.

03. Place the avocado cut into pieces into a food processor and add the egg yolks, mayonnaise, lemon juice, salt and pepper. Process until smooth. Alternatively, mash with a fork until creamy and well combined.

04. Enjoy with cucumber slices and spring onion on top, or ... fill up the egg white halves and make deviled eggs. To avoid browning, store in an airtight container and keep for up to 5 days.

## NUTRITION:

Net carbs 1.1 g

Protein 2.2 g

Fat 14.8 g

Calories 148 kcal

Total carbs 2.5 g

Fiber 1.4 g

Sugars 0.3 g

Saturated Fat 2.7 g

Sodium 263 mg (11% RDA)

Magnesium 8 mg (2% RDA)

Potassium 141 mg (7% EMR)

# KETO ROLLUPS

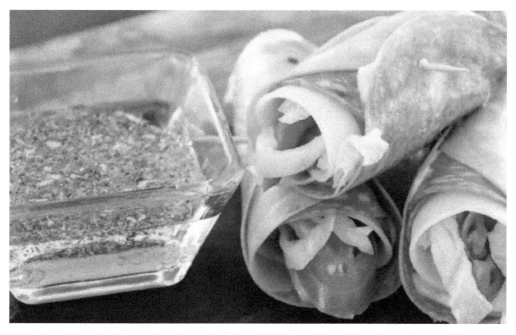

High fat, Keto Italian sub roll-up lunch with 20g of fat, 10g of protein and less than 1 net carb. The perfect Keto lunch.

SERVINGS: 4

**INGREDIENTS:**

4 Slices Genoa Salami

4 Slices Mortadella

4 Slices Sopressata

4 Slices Pepperoni

4 Slices Provolone omit for dairy-free option Paleo Lime Mayo or store-bough mayo we love Chosen Foods Avocado Oil Mayo Shredded Lettuce

Extra toppings our favorites are banana peppers, jalapeño peppers, roasted red peppers, and black olives, if desired

Avocado Oil or Olive Oil

Apple Cider Vinegar

Italian Seasoning

Toothpicks

## DIRECTIONS:

01. Layer the meat slices from largest to smallest. For the brand we use (Boar's Head), the order is: – Genoa Salami – Mortadella – Sopressata – Pepperoni

02. Spread a thin layer of mayo on the stack, making sure to leave space at the top of the largest piece to keep it from squishing out when you roll them up.

03. Add a slice of provolone on top of the mayo, about halfway from the top. Add a small handful of lettuce to the lower half and top with desired toppings (optional).

04. Have the toothpicks nearby and ready to grab. Starting from the bottom of the cheese, gently

05. When you get to the end, secure the outer meat edges with a toothpick.

06. To serve, pour 2 parts oil and 1 part vinegar into a small dipping ramekin. Sprinkle some Italian seasoning on top. Dip the roll-ups in the oil/vinegar and enjoy!

07. Store extras in the fridge, wrapped individually in plastic wrap, for up to a week. These make for delicious and easy school lunches.

## NUTRITION:

Calories 234.3 kcal

Carbohydrates 0.9 g

Protein 10 g

Fat 20.6 g

# CREAM CHEESE COOKIES

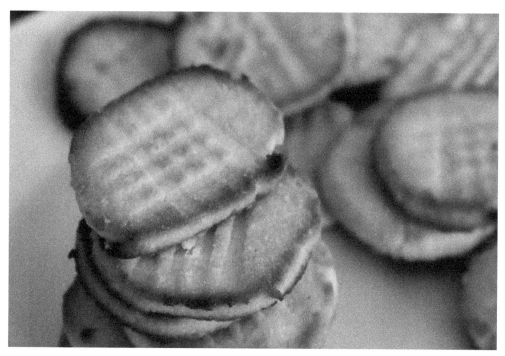

Low carb cookies baked with cream cheese and coconut flour

SERVINGS: 15 COOKIES

## INGREDIENTS:

½ cup Coconut Flour

3 Tbsp Cream cheese softened

1 Egg

½ cup Butter softened

½ cup Erythritol or other sugar substitute

1 tsp Vanilla extract

½ tsp baking powder

¼ tsp salt

## DIRECTIONS:

01. In a bowl, cream together the butter, cream cheese and erythritol (or sugar substitute of choice).

02. Add the vanilla extra and egg. Beat until smooth.

03. Add the coconut flour, baking powder and salt and beat until combined. The mixture will be sticky.

04. Place the mixture onto a piece of wax paper (or parchment paper). Mould into a log shape, using the paper to roll out and wrap the paper around the dough and secure the ends like a Christmas cracker.

05. Place in the fridge to firm up for at least an hour.

06. Preheat the oven to 180C/350F degrees.

07. Line a baking tray with parchment paper.

08. Remove the dough from the fridge and cut into 1 cm slices.

09. Place the slices on the baking tray.

10. Bake for 15-18 minutes until golden.


## NUTRITION:

Calories 91 kcal

Carbohydrates 3 g

Protein 1 g

Fat 8 g

Fiber 2 g

Net Carbs 1 g

# GRILLED CHEESE SANDWICH

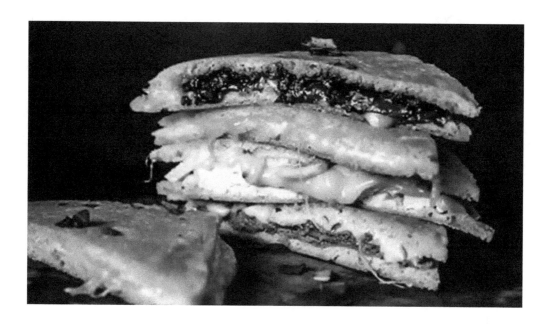

There is nothing quite so satisfying as picking up a big, melty slice of grilled cheese sandwich and biting into that melt goodness. Especially when it's low-carb!

## INGREDIENTS:

¼ cup almond flour (25 g/ 0.9 oz)

½ tsp gluten-free baking powder

1 Tbsp light olive oil or extra virgin olive oil (15 ml) pinch of sea salt

1 large egg


Filling: 1 slice cheddar cheese (28 g/ 1 oz)

1 slice Swiss cheese (28 g/ 1 oz)

Optional variations (use instead of the above filling): 2 Tbsp Red Eye Bacon Jam,

2-3 slices Brie cheese and handful of spinach

3-4 oz cooked chicken,

¼ sliced avocado,

1-2 slices Jarlsburg cheese

1-2 slices Pastrami,

3-4 slices Provolone cheese and 2 slices red onion

## DIRECTIONS:

01. Place all of the bread ingredients into a small bowl and mix well.

02. Grease a ramekin, or like me find a bread-shaped storage container. Pour the mixture into the container and shake to distribute evenly.

03. Microwave on high for 90 seconds. Turn out and cool on a rack. Note: If you don't have a microwave, you can use the oven. Preheat to 175 °C/ 350 °F and bake for 12-15 minutes or until cooked through.

04. When cool, cut in half and spread with butter, if desired. Place the cheese slices in the middle and toast for approx. 5 minutes (or try any of our suggested variations).

05. Eat with gusto. Store, wrapped, in the refrigerator for up to 2 days.

## NUTRITION:

Net carbs 4.3 g

Protein 25.6 g

Fat 49.4 g

Calories 564 kcal

Total carbs 6.8 g

Fiber 2.5 g

Sugars 1.5 g

Saturated fat 14.8 g

Sodium 761 mg (33% RDA)

Magnesium 90 mg (23% RDA)

Potassium 276 mg (14% EMR)

# LOW-CARB BACON JAM

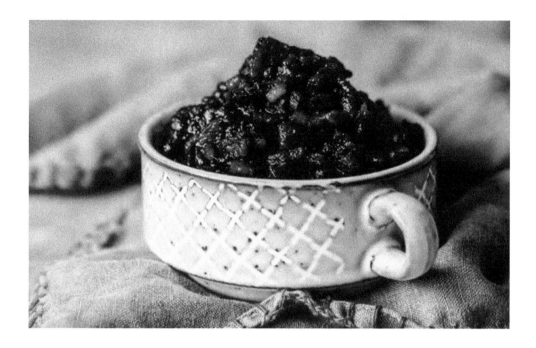

## INGREDIENTS:

500 g bacon slices (1.1 lb)

1 large red onion (150 g/ 5.3 oz)

½ cup Sukrin Gold or Swerve (80 g/ 2.8 oz)

½ cup strong black coffee (120 ml/ 4 fl oz)

¼ cup water (60 ml/ 2 fl oz)

2 Tbsp balsamic vinegar (30 ml) - avoid extra sweet thick balsamic vinegar

1 Tbsp coconut aminos (15 ml)

## DIRECTIONS:

01. Cut the bacon into small strips. Peel and slice the onion. Prepare the coffee and set aside. 02. Cook the sliced bacon in a skillet until cooked but not crispy.

03. Remove bacon from pan and place in a bowl to set aside. To the same pan where you cooked the bacon add sliced red onion and mix until covered in the rendered bacon grease. Cook until onion is softened, approx. 5 minutes.

04. Add the Sukrin Gold, stir through and then cook on low heat for 15 minutes until

the onions are caramelised.

05. Return the bacon to the skillet and add the coffee and water. Cook on medium-high for 30 minutes, stirring regularly.

06. Stir the balsamic vinegar and coconut aminos through and cook for a further couple of minutes.

07. Allow to cool slightly and then spoon into jars. Serve with keto bread and sliced cheese such as brie, manchego or hard goat cheese.

08. Store sealed in the refrigerator for up to 2 weeks.

## NUTRITION:

Net carbs 1.2 g

Protein 4.4 g

Fat 7.9 g

Calories 94 kcal

Total carbs 1.3 g

Fiber 0.1 g

Sugars 0.9 g

Saturated fat 2.6 g

Sodium 264 mg (11% RDA)

Magnesium 5 mg (1% RDA)

Potassium 85 mg (4% EMR)

# BACON "CHIPS" AND GUACAMOLE DIP

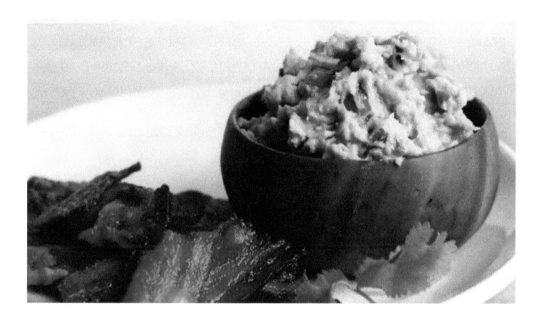

Swap tortilla chips for crisp bacon "chips" and dip in rich guacamole till your heart's content! TOOLS Baking sheet, Parchment paper, Small bowl

## INGREDIENTS:

8-10 strips thick-cut, pasture-raised bacon

2 avocados

¼ cup red onion, chopped

1 Tbsp cilantro, chopped

1 Tbsp jalapeño, minced

¼ tsp ground cumin

¼ tsp sea salt

## DIRECTIONS:

01. Preheat oven to 375°F and line a baking sheet with parchment paper.

02. Slice each bacon strip into 2-3 inch pieces and lay on the baking sheet. Bake 15-20 minutes. Remove from the oven and allow the bacon to crisp up on a plate.

03. In a small bowl, use a fork to mash the avocados. Stir in the red onion, jalapeño, ground cumin and sea salt.

04. Serve bacon chips alongside the guacamole dip.

## NUTRITION:

Protein 14 g

Carbohydrates 4 g

Fat 21 g

# AVOCADO EGG SALAD

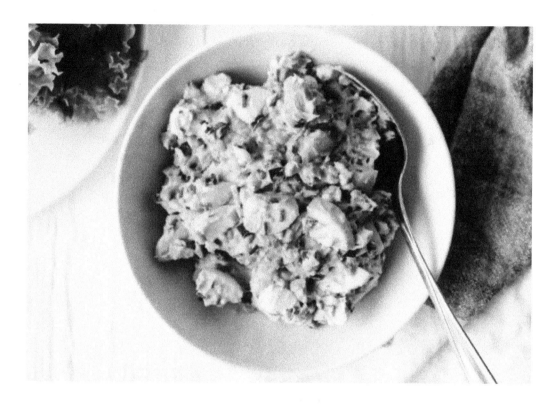

This healthy egg salad is made extra creamy from the addition of avocado. Such a tasty twist on the traditional egg salad. The nutrition information is for the egg salad only and doesn't include info on lettuce if you choose to make lettuce wraps with this.

SERVING: 6

## INGREDIENTS:

6 boiled eggs

2 avocado, diced

½ lemon

¼ cup minced red onion

2 tsp fresh dill

½ tsp salt

½ tsp pepper

## DIRECTIONS:

01. Peel and dice the boiled eggs and place in a medium mixing bowl.

02. Add the avocado to the eggs and stir well. The avocado will become creamier the more you stir and coat the eggs.

03. Squeeze the lemon half over the eggs and stir in the onion, dill, salt, and pepper. Stir well to combine the mixture.

04. Serve immediately.

## NUTRITION:

Calories 160

Total Fat 12 g

 Saturated Fat 3g

Trans Fat 0 g

Unsaturated Fat 8 g

Cholesterol 187 mg

Sodium 242 mg

Carbohydrates 6 g

Fiber 3 g

Sugar 1 g

Protein 7 g

# KETO AVOCADO TOAST RECIPE WITH PISTACHIO AND TOMATO

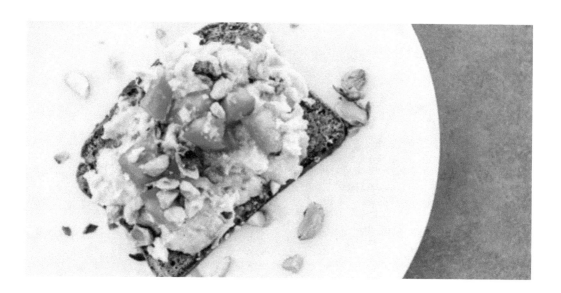

YIELD: 1 SERVING

**INGREDIENTS:** 1 slice of Keto bread, toasted

½ ripe avocado

½ tsp lime juice

⅛ Tomato, dice

6 pistachios, crushed

Sea salt to taste

2 tsp (10 ml) extra virgin olive oil

**NUTRITION:**

Calories 376

Sugar 1 g

Fat 38 g

Carbohydrates 11 g

Fiber 8 g

Protein 5 g

## DIRECTIONS:

01. Toast a slice of Keto bread.

02. Cut the avocado in half and drizzle the lime juice over it.

03. Place the avocado half on top of the toast and smash it into the toast.

04. Sprinkle the diced tomatoes, crushed pistachios, and sea salt over the avocado.

05. Drizzle extra virgin olive oil over the avocado toast.

06. Enjoy with a knife and fork or using your hands.

# TASTY FETA BURGERS (EGG-FREE)

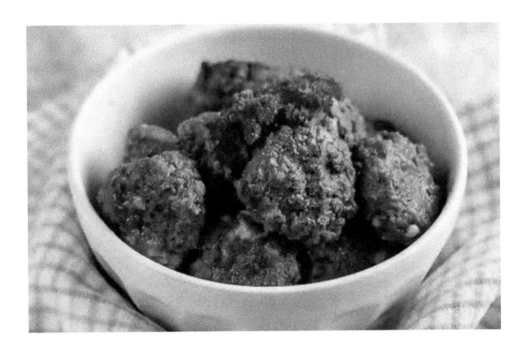

## INGREDIENTS:

14 oz (400 g) organic ground beef

4 oz (115 g) crumbled organic feta cheese

2 tsp dried organic oregano

2 organic garlic cloves, peeled and crushed

2 oz (60 g) organic full-fat plain Greek yogurt

## NUTRITION:

Protein 24.2 g

Fat 17.3 g

Net carbs 0.9 g

Calories 256 kcal

## DIRECTIONS:

01. Combine all ingredients in a large bowl. Mix well with clean hands until the mixture is well mixed. This takes a couple of minutes.

02. Form into patties of your preferred size.

03. Cook the patties in a skillet in butter or in olive oil. You can also grill them. Don't cook too long, only until the patties are just cooked through. Otherwise they might turn out dry.

# KETO CRACK CHICKEN

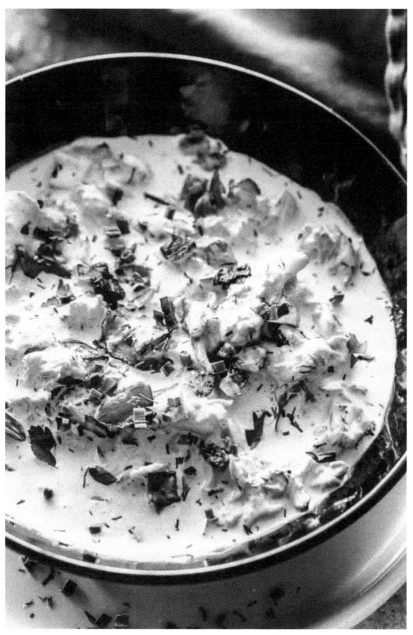

Rich, creamy, and full of flavor, this Keto Instant Pot Crack Chicken Recipe is sure to be a favorite family dinner.

**SERVES:** 8 SERVINGS (YIELDS ABOUT 7 CUPS TOTAL

## INGREDIENTS:

2 slices bacon, chopped

2 lbs (910 g) boneless, skinless chicken breasts

2 (8 oz/227 g) blocks cream cheese

½ cup (120 ml) water

2 Tbsp apple cider vinegar

1 Tbsp dried chives

1½ tsp garlic powder

1½ tsp onion powder

1 tsp crushed red pepper flakes

1 tsp dried dill

¼ tsp salt

¼ tsp black pepper

½ cup (2 oz/57 g) shredded cheddar

1 scallion, green and white parts, thinly sliced

## NUTRITION:

Calories 437

Fat 27.6

Potassium 390

Net Carbs 4.3

Carbohydrates 4.5

Sodium 420

Fiber 0.2

Protein 41.2

## DIRECTIONS:

01. Turn pressure cooker on, press "Sauté", and wait 2 minutes for the pot to heat up. Add the chopped bacon and cook until crispy. Transfer to a plate and set aside. Press "Cancel" to stop sautéing.

02. Add the chicken, cream cheese, water, vinegar, chives, garlic powder, onion powder, crushed red pepper flakes, dill, salt, and black pepper to the pot. Turn the pot on Manual, High Pressure for 15 minutes and then do a quick release.

03. Use tongs to transfer the chicken to a large plate, shred it with 2 forks, and return it back to the pot.

04. Stir in the cheddar cheese.

05. Top with the crispy bacon and scallion, and serve.

# TOMATO FETA SOUP

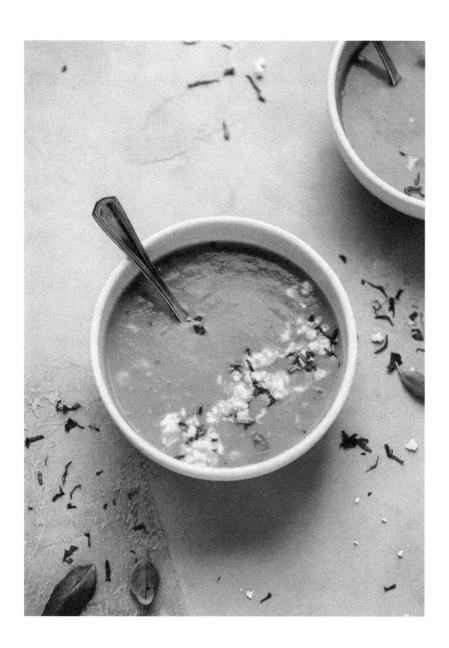

**INGREDIENTS:**

2 Tbsp olive oil or butter

¼ cup chopped onion

2 cloves garlic

½ tsp salt

⅛ tsp black pepper

1 tsp pesto sauce — optional

½ tsp dried oregano

1 tsp dried basil

1 Tbsp tomato paste — optional 10 tomatoes, skinned, seeded and chopped — or two 14.5 oz cans of peeled tomatoes

1 tsp honey, sugar or erythritol — optional

3 cups water

⅓ Cup heavy cream

⅔ Cup feta cheese — crumbled

## DIRECTIONS:

01. Heat olive oil (butter) over medium heat in a large pot (Dutch Oven). Add the onion and cook for 2 minutes, stirring frequently. Add the garlic and cook for 1 minute. Add tomatoes, salt, pepper, pesto (optional), oregano, basil, tomato paste and water. Bring to a boil, then reduce to a simmer. Add sweetener.

02. Cook on medium heat for 20 minutes, until the tomatoes are tender and cooker. Using an immersion blender, blend until smooth. Add the cream and feta cheese. Cook for 1 more minute.

03. Add more salt if needed. Serve warm.

## NUTRITION:

Calories 170

Fat 13 g

Saturated Fat 8 g

Cholesterol 43 mg

Sodium 464 mg

Potassium 542 mg

Carbohydrates 10 g

Fiber 2 g

Sugar 6 g

Protein 4 g

# LOW CARB GREEN SMOOTHIE

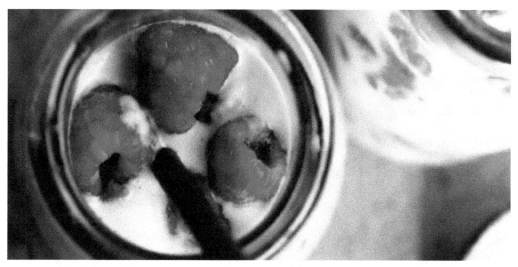

This delicious and nutrient dense low carb green smoothie recipe tastes like a milkshake without the carbs! Most delicious and healthy way to start the day!

SERVINGS: 2

## INGREDIENTS:

½ Avocado

1 cup Spinach

1 scoop Low Carb Protein Powder Vanilla

½ cup Low Carb Milk

5-6 Leaves Mint

Lemon Juice optional

**NUTRITION:**

Calories 150 kcal

 Carbohydrates 5 g

Protein 14 g

Fat 8 g

Saturated Fat 1 g

Cholesterol 30 mg

Sodium 135 mg

Potassium 388 mg

Fiber 3 g

 Sugar 1 g

## DIRECTIONS:

01. Add INGREDIENTS: to a blender + blend! If you'd like to eat this as a smoothie bowl, add 2 cups of ice.

02. Add your toppings and enjoy!

# KETO PROTEIN SHAKE

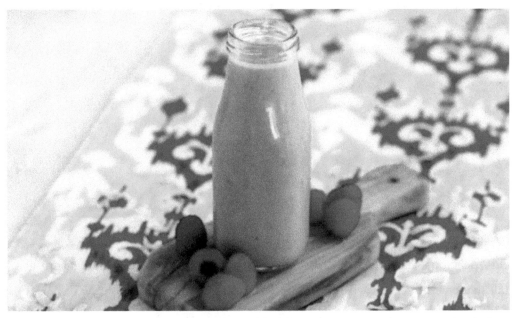

Add a dose of protein to your morning with this sweet, creamy keto protein shake—with NO protein powder! Collagen powder is a cleaner alternative to most protein powders, with incredible joint, hair, and nail benefits. You won't taste it, but your body will appreciate the nutritious boost!

## INGREDIENTS:

1 cup coconut milk

⅓ cup frozen raspberries

1 Tbspcoconut oil

1 scoop collagen sweetener of choice, to taste

## DIRECTIONS:

01. Add all ingredients to a blender and blend until smooth.

02. Serve and enjoy! Yields 1 keto protein shake.

## NUTRITION:

Calories 549

Sugar 6 g

Fat 50 g

Carbohydrates 10 g

Net Carbs per Serving 7 g

Fiber 3 g

Protein 10 g

# KETO GREEN SMOOTHIE

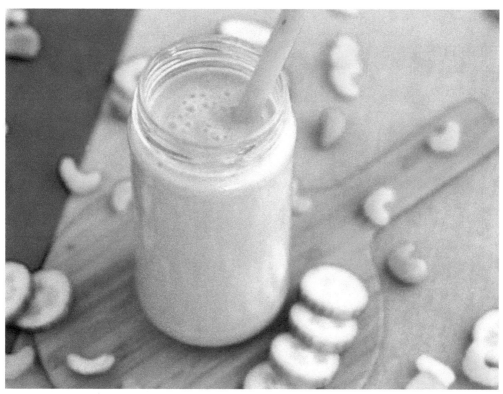

This vibrant keto green smoothie is loaded with color, nutrients, and veggies! Cucumber and celery create a refreshing flavor burst, while the avocado and cashew milk keep the texture silky-smooth. With a dash of energizing MCTs, it's a simple, sippable low carb breakfast to fuel your morning!

YIELD: 1 SERVING

## INGREDIENTS:

½ cup cashew milk

1 baby cucumber

1 stalkcelery

½ avocado

1 Tbspcoconut oil

1 tsp matcha powder sweetener of choice, to taste

## DIRECTIONS:

01. Add all ingredients to a blender and blend until smooth.

02. Serve and enjoy

## NUTRITION:

Calories 278

Sugar 2 g

Fat 27 g

Carbohydrates 12 g

Net Carbs per Serving 6 g

Fiber 6 g

Protein 3 g

# ANTI-INFLAMMATORY GOLDEN MILK KETO SMOOTHIE

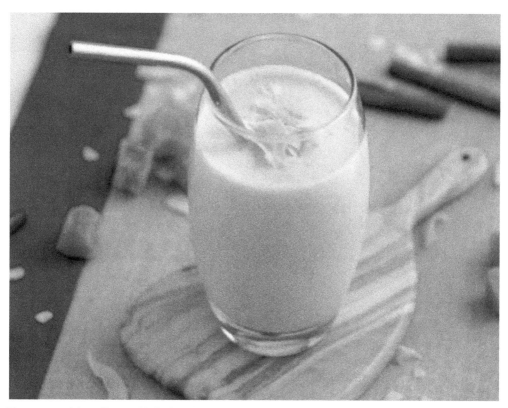

For an exciting flavor kick AND a super food boost, try this anti-inflammatory golden milk smoothie! It's made with 2 of the most powerful anti-inflammatory foods on Earth: turmeric & ginger. Blend it up with frozen coconut milk cubes for an ultra-creamy keto smoothie that's rich in wholesome fats— with just 4g net carbs!

YIELD: 1 SERVING

**INGREDIENTS:**

6-8 coconut milk ice cubes, thawed slightly (or ~1 cup coconut milk)

1-2 Tbsp additional coconut milk or water

½ tsp vanilla

1 Tbspcoconut oil

½ tsp turmeric

¼ tsp cinnamon

Pinch of ground ginger

Pinch of salt

Sweetener of choice to taste

## DIRECTIONS:

01. Add all ingredients to a blender and blend until smooth.

 02. Serve and enjoy!

03. Yields 1 keto smoothie.


To make coconut milk ice cubes:

01. Shake can of coconut milk, blend the milk, or whisk well until smooth with no clumps.

02. Pour into ice cube tray and freeze 3-4 hours, or overnight.


## NUTRITION:

Calories 492

 Sugar 3 g

Fat 50 g

Carbohydrates 4 g

 Net Carbs per Serving 4 g

 Fiber 0 g

Protein 0 g

# CINNAMON ALMOND BULLETPROOF KETO SHAKE

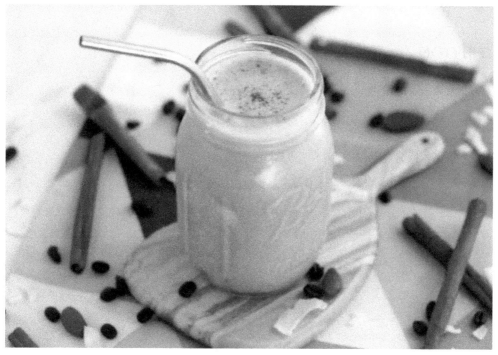

Get your coffee AND on-the-go breakfast all in one cup with this Bulletproof ketogenic shake! Frozen coconut milk cubes add creaminess and nutritious fats, without watering down your coffee. Every cinnamon-y sip of this low carb shake is so satisfying, energizing, and packed with fats for fuel!

YIELD: 1 SERVING

**INGREDIENTS:**

1 cup coffee

 3-4 coconut milk ice cubes (or ~⅓-½ cup coconut milk)

1 Tbspcoconut oil or MCT oil

2 Tbspalmond butter

1 Tbspflax meal

½ tsp cinnamon sweetener of choice, to taste

Pinch of salt

## DIRECTIONS:

01. Add all ingredients to a blender and blend until smooth.

02. Serve and enjoy! Yields 1 Bulletproof keto shake.

## NUTRITION:

Calories 503

Sugar 3 g

Fat 49 g

Carbohydrates 11 g

Net Carbs per Serving 6 g

Fiber 5 g

Protein 9 g

# BUFFALO CHICKEN JALAPENO POPPERS

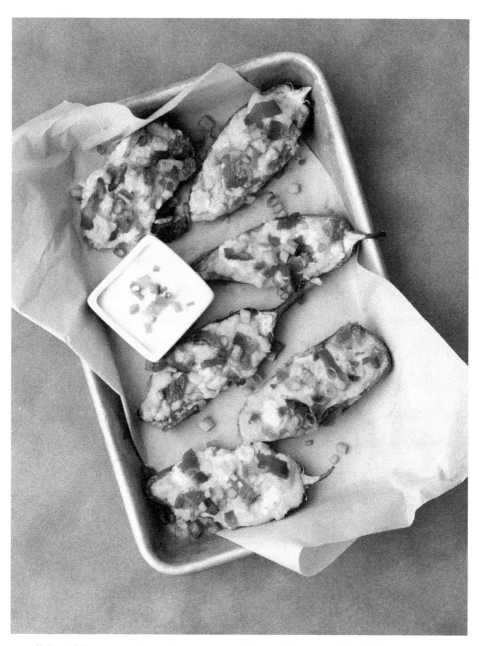

Two traditional bar appetizers just got a major makeover with this recipe. How about instead of choosing between jalapeno poppers or buffalo chicken wings, you just get both in one dish? Talk about a match made in heaven. Add some creamy ranch or blue cheese dressing on the side, and you are good to go!

SERVINGS: 5-4

## INGREDIENTS:

30 large jalapeño peppers, halved lengthwise and seeded

24 oz ground chicken

6 cloves garlic, minced

1 ½ tsp onion powder

1 ½ tsp fine sea salt

12 oz cream cheese (1 ½ cup), softened

1 ½ cup crumbled blue cheese, divided

¾ cup shredded mozzarella cheese

¾ cup buffalo wing sauce

12 strips bacon, cooked crisp and crumbled

6 green onions, sliced, for garnish

Ranch dressing, for serving

## NUTRITION:

Calories 252

Fat 19 g

Carbohydrates 4.6 g

Fiber 1 g

Protein 16 g

## DIRECTIONS:

01. Preheat the oven to 350°F. Line a rimmed baking sheet with a silicone baking mat or parchment paper. Spread the jalapeño halves across the baking sheet.

02. Heat a large skillet over medium heat. To the skillet, add the chicken, garlic, onion powder, and sea salt. Sauté until the chicken is no longer pink and is cooked all the way through.

03. Transfer the cooked chicken to a large mixing bowl and add the cream cheese, ¼ cup of the blue cheese crumbles, mozzarella cheese, and Buffalo wing sauce. Mix until all of the ingredients are well combined.

04. Fill each jalapeno with a mound of the chicken mixture. Top with the remaining ¼ cup of blue cheese crumbles and bacon.

05. Bake for 30 minutes, until the top is golden brown.

06. Top with green onions before serving.

CPSIA information can be obtained
at www.ICGtesting.com
Printed in the USA
BVHW011627110321
602276BV00011B/1028

9 781801 724661